Raja Jouini
Imen Helal
Sarra yacoub

Diagnosis of Hirschsprung's disease

Raja Jouini
Imen Helal
Sarra yacoub

Diagnosis of Hirschsprung's disease

Study of the diagnostic performance of the anti-calretinin antibody.

ScienciaScripts

Cover image: www.ingimage.com

This book is a translation from the original published under ISBN 978-620-6-72985-3.

Publisher:
Sciencia Scripts
is a trademark of
Dodo Books Indian Ocean Ltd. and OmniScriptum S.R.L publishing group

120 High Road, East Finchley, London, N2 9ED, United Kingdom
Str. Armeneasca 28/1, office 1, Chisinau MD-2012, Republic of Moldova, Europe
Managing Directors: Ieva Konstantinova, Victoria Ursu
info@omniscriptum.com

Printed at: see last page
ISBN: 978-620-8-62439-2

TABLE OF CONTENTS

INTRODUCTION

Hirschsprung's disease (HD) is a rare congenital disorder defined by absence of total of ganglion cells (GC) in the meyenteric plexuses of Meissner's submucosa and Auerbach'muscularis, beginning at the anal sphincter and extending over a variable part of the digestive tract [1]. Its prevalence varies from 1 to 1.63 per 10,000 births. Once always fatal, surgical treatment has reduced mortality from the disease to 3% in developed countries [2,3]. MH affects newborns. It causes non-specific symptoms, including chronic constipation and neonatal obstruction [4]. Radiological examination helps to determine the extent of the disease by identifying the presumed transition zone (PTZ) that separates the healthy ganglionic intestinal segment from the aganglionic intestinal segment [5,6]. Diagnosis is histopathological and requires precision as to the integrity of the surgical boundary. It is based on staining of slides with haematein-eosin and, in most reference centres, on enzyme-linked immunosorbent assays of acetylcholinesterase activity [7-9]. Histopathological examination is performed on rectal biopsies taken from presumed diseased areas (PDAs) for diagnostic purposes and from presumed healthy areas (PHAs) and PTAs during extemporaneous examinations to guide the surgical procedure[3,5]. Histopathological examination poses difficulties in certain cases. CGs are immature in newborns and can be confused with other cells [4]. In other , their detection can be laborious, requiring use of several levels of tissue block section to prove with certainty the total absence of GCs[10]. In addition, histopathological examination involves superficial rectal biopsies, devoid of muscularis and therefore not including Auerbach's plexuses in 9 to 17% of cases. These situations lead to inconclusive results and diagnostic delays, often with serious consequences [11-13]. Enzyme-linked immunosorbent assay using acetylcholinesterase reveals extrinsic nerve net hyperplasia, which is the second characteristic histological sign of HD. However, this method is still limited to certain paediatric reference centres [13]. To remedy the shortcomings of histopathological and enzyme-linked immunosorbent assays on biopsy samples, a number of teams have begun looking for biomarkers of HD [14]. Many studies have focused on markers of the enteral nervous system, in particular calretinin, a vitamin D-dependent protein that binds and buffers intracellular calcium [1,7,10,12,14]. The disappearance of calretinin in digestive tracts affected by HD was described in 2004 [15]. The use an antibody directed against calretinin and the evaluation of the performance of this marker in the diagnosis of HD has since been the subject of numerous studies [1,7,10,12,14]. The aim of our work was to evaluate the diagnostic performance of the anti-calretinin antibody on biopsy samples taken in the context of suspected MH.

METHODS

1. Type study

This was a retrospective study of all biopsies performed in patients followed at the paediatric surgery department of Habib Thameur Hospital for suspected MH between December 1995 and September 2017. These biopsies were sent to the Department of Pathological Anatomy and Cytology at Habib Thameur Hospital. They were indexed from the department's register of anatomopathological reports. We began by reviewing all the biopsies taken. This review was carried out by a senior pathologist and was then used as a reference test in the study of the diagnostic performance of the anti-calretinin antibody.

2. Case selection criteria

2.1. INCLUSION CRITERIA

All biopsies taken during the study period and sent for suspicion of HD, whatever the definitive clinical diagnosis.

2.2. Exclusion

▶ Patients whose medical records were unavailable

▶ Cases for which no information on the sampling zone (SPA, MPA or PTZ) could be found, either in the pathology reports or in the medical records. total of 127 patients with suspected HD were identified during the study period, of whom 47 cases were excluded for the following reasons (Figure 1):

▶ Unavailability of medical records (40)

▶ No mention of the sampling area (7)

Thus, patients who met the selection criteria and were selected to do the subject of our study were 80.

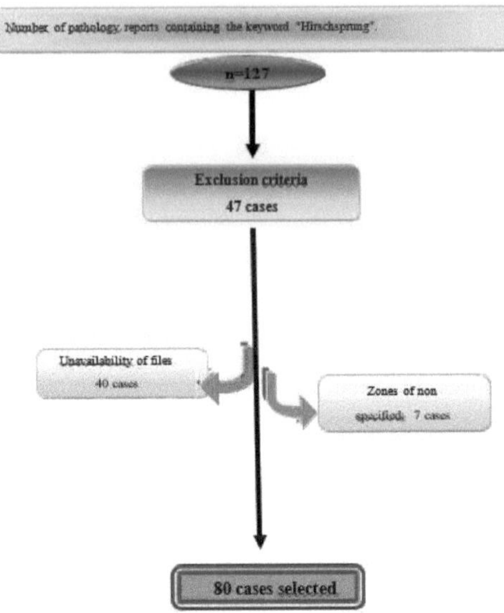

Figure 1: Case selection summary diagram

3. Data collection

3.1. Clinical data

The following clinical and epidemiological parameters were recorded in the files:

- ▶ The scope of MH
- ▶ The genre
- ▶ Inbreeding
- ▶ Family history
- ▶ Associated malformations
- ▶ Circumstances of discovery :

– meconium emission

– Chronic constipation or intestinal obstruction

▶ The operating procedure

▶ The extent of Hirschsprung's disease was assessed on the basis of :

- The limits of the surgical resections mentioned on the operative reports and verified on the anatomopathological reports.
- The size of the colonic resection specimens, correlated with the patient's age, when the level of resection was not mentioned in the operative and pathological reports.

3.2. Data from radiological and functional investigations

▶ Results of the barium enema

▶ Results of anorectal manometry

3.3. Anatomopathological data

3.3.1. Macroscopic data

The presumed harvesting zones were identified. These were SPAs, ZPTs and ZPMs.

3.3.2. Histopathological data

The samples sent for clinical suspicion of MH were distributed as follows:

▶ Pre-operative surgical biopsies, taken under general anaesthetic, to confirm or refute the diagnosis.

▶ Intraoperative biopsies are taken for extemporaneous examination to identify the healthy zone.

The samples included in our study were fixed in 10% diluted formalin and then included in paraffin and the tissue slides were stained with haematein-eosin. The slides re-read for both pre-operative and intra-operative biopsies and were performed blindly without knowledge of the initial diagnosis. The anatomopathological parameters assessed were as follows:

▶ The depth of the biopsy, specifying which layers of the wall were removed

▶ Presence or absence of GCs. The latter have been defined as polygonal cells with abundant eosinophilic cytoplasm, an eccentric nucleus and a large nucleolus [16].

▶ The presence or absence of nerve hyperplasia. Nerve hyperplasia, was defined from a diameter greater than 40 μm, based on data from the literature [14]

▶ The number of levels of tissue blocks cut and the number of slides studied for each case

▶ Special colourings carried out (type and number)

3.3.3. Immunohistochemical data

3.3.3.1. Technical data

The selection of samples was based on :

▶ Pre-operative biopsies

▶ Intraoperative sampling when the preoperative biopsy was not performed

The immunohistochemical study was carried out using the ready-to-use mouse monoclonal anti-calretinin antibody "Bond TM calretinin cal6". The various stages of the immunohistochemical reaction were automated (Leica BOND-MAX).

3.3.3.2. Interpretation of the results of the immunohistochemical study

Immunohistochemistry slides were read blindly without knowledge of the

diagnosis made initially or on re-reading. The various elements assessed were :

▶ Cytoplasmic and nuclear labelling of GCs

▶ Marking of interstitial nerve fibres present in the chorion, tunica muscularis mucosa and submucosa

▶ Granular marking of nerve nets

Mast cells and mesothelial cells were used as internal controls.

4. Statistical analysis

The data was entered using SPSS® (Statistical Package for Social Science) version 21 software. For the descriptive analysis, we calculated frequencies and percentages for the qualitative variables and averages for quantitative variables. For the analytical study, only samples taken in MPAs that confirmed or refuted the diagnosis were included. Cohen's kappa test (K) was used to analyse concordance. The results were evaluated using the cut-off values in Table I.

Table I: Interpretation of the kappa coefficient

K	Estimation of the degree of
0,8 à 1	Excellent
0,6 à 0,8	Good
0,4 à 0,6	Medium
0,2 à 0,4	Low
0 à 0,2	Negligible
<0	Bad

The immunohistochemical study using the anti-calretinin antibody was studied as the diagnostic test to be evaluated by calculating its sensitivity, specificity, negative predictive value and positive predictive value. criteria for positive labelling with anti-calretinin antibody were those reported in the literature [6,14,15], i.e. the presence of at least one of the following elements:

- ▶ Labelling of cytoplasmic and nuclear GCs
- ▶ Marking of interstitial nerve fibres in the chorion, muscularis mucosae or submucosa

The diagnosis of MH was made if immunohistochemical staining was negative.

RESULTS

1. DESCRIPTIVE STUDY

1.1. DIAGNOSIS OF HIRSCHSPRUNG'S DISEASE IN THE STUDY POPULATION

Of the 80 patients included in our study, 69 (84%) were diagnosed with HD on the basis of histopathological data from preoperative and intraoperative biopsies. Among the 11 remaining cases, the diagnosis of HD was invalidated by histopathological study of the pre-operative biopsies in 10/11 cases (91%). In the last case, despite a histopathological diagnosis of MH made on the pre-operative biopsy in the absence of GC, the good clinical evolution did not allow this diagnosis to be retained.

1.2. EPIDEMIOLOGICAL DATA

1.2.1. THE GENRE

Of the 69 patients in whom the diagnosis of HD was suspected, there was a clear male predominance, with a sex ratio (boys/girls) of 3.6 (Figure 2).

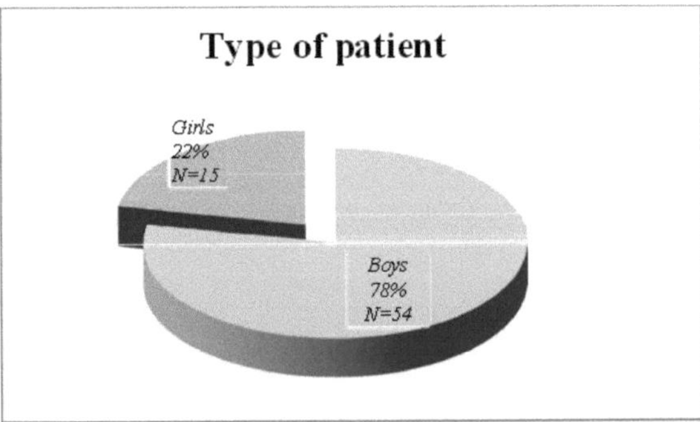

Figure 2: Distribution of the population with Hirshsprung's disease by gender

1.2.2. AGE

The mean age of the 69 patients with HD was 555 days, or 18 months and 15 days, with extremes of 1 day and 15 years. MH appeared before age of 2 in 68 cases (99%) and at the age of 15 in only one. cases (Figure 3).

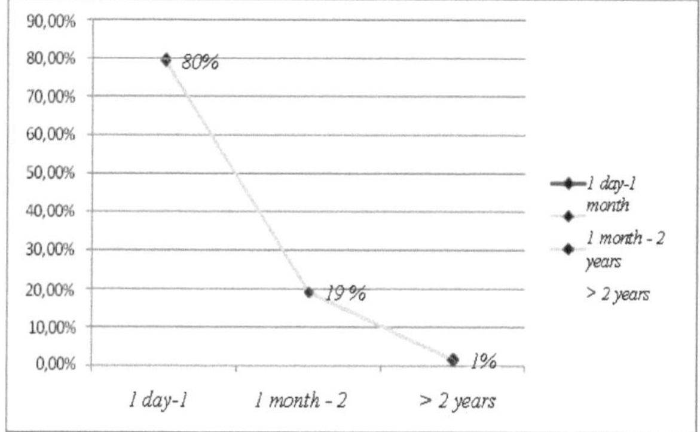

Figure 3:Distribution of age of onset of symptoms in the study population with Hirschsprung's disease

1.3. CLINICAL DATA

1.3.1. HOW HIRSCHSPRUNG'S DISEASE IS DISCOVERED

MH was revealed by (Figure 4):

- Acute intestinal obstruction in 49 cases (71%)
- Chronic constipation since birth in 31 cases (45%)
- Delayed meconium output in 40 cases. This symptom was reported in only 57 cases (70%).

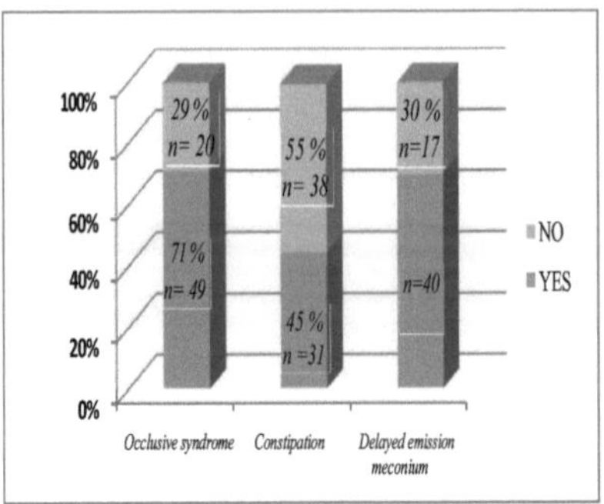

Figure 4: Signs of Hirschsprung's disease in 69 patients with the disease

1.3.2. The extent of Hirschsprung's disease

The 68 patients operated on included :

- 20 rectal forms (29%)
- 37 sigmoid forms (54%)
- Eight left colic forms (12%)
- A total colonic form (2%)
- Two forms extending to the ileum (3%)

The classic forms (rectal and sigmoidal) were more frequently observed boys than in girls (Figure 5).

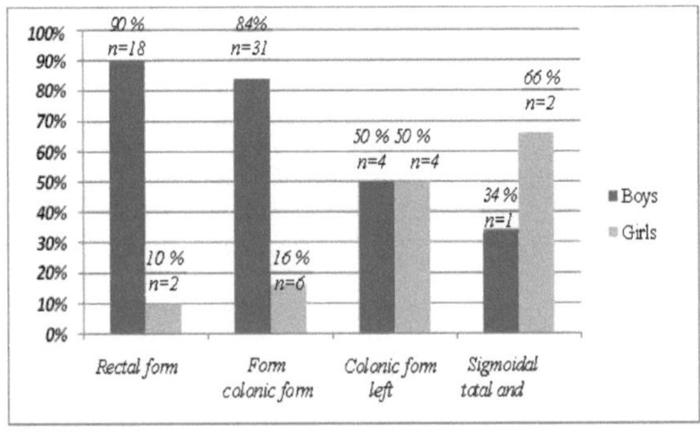

Figure 5: Gender distribution of the extent of Hirschsprung's disease in operated patients.

1.3.3. Family background

A family history neonatal enteropathy was reported in 2 of 69 patients. MH carriers (3%):

▶ A 2-year-old patient whose paternal uncle had a congenital enteropathy, the exact nature of which could not be determined.

▶ A case MH in twin sisters a left colic form and a right colic form. of a total colonic form.

1.3.4. Consanguinitis

Consanguinity was noted in the medical records in 3 cases. These were first-degree consanguinity in one case and two cases of 2th degree consanguinity.

1.3.5. Associated signs

Twenty-two patients with HD had associated congenital anomalies. The congenital anomaly most frequently observed in our study was umbilical hernia, followed by Trisomy 21 (Table II). One case was a Waardenburg syndrome combining facial dysmorphia, skin hyperpigmentation of the limbs and sensorineural deafness.

Table II: Distribution of congenital malformations by gender

Associated congenital malformations		Typ e		Number of cases
	Male		Female	
Umbilical hernia	10		4	14
Unilateral renal agenesis and vesicoureteral reflux	0		1	1
Vesico-ureteral reflux	1		0	1
Mega-ureter	1		0	1
Pyeloureteral junction syndrome	1		0	1
Trisomy 21	2		1	3
Waardenburg syndrome	1		0	1

1.4. Radiological and functional examination data

1.4.1. Barium enema

Barium enema was performed in 69 out of 80 patients

Sixty-three of these patients were carriers of HD (91%) and six were disease-free.

ZPT was identified in 43 of 63 patients with MH (68%). It identified in :

- ▶ Rectum in 11/43 cases (26%)
- ▶ From the recto-sigmoid area in 25/43 cases (58%)
- ▶ Left colon in 7/43 cases (16%) Of the remaining 20 enemas :
- ▶ Fourteen enemas (70%) showed dilatation or an abnormality in the length of the colon with no disparity in calibre.
- ▶ Six enemas were normal (30%)

Opaque enemas from patients without MH showed rectal ZPT 2 cases and recto-colic dilatation without disparity in calibre in 4 cases.

1.4.2. Anorectal manometry

Anorectal manometry was performed in 50/80 patients (). The inhibitory recto-anal reflex (IRAR) was absent in 37 of 44 patients with a MH (84%) and in 4 of 6 MH-free patients (71%) (Figure 6).

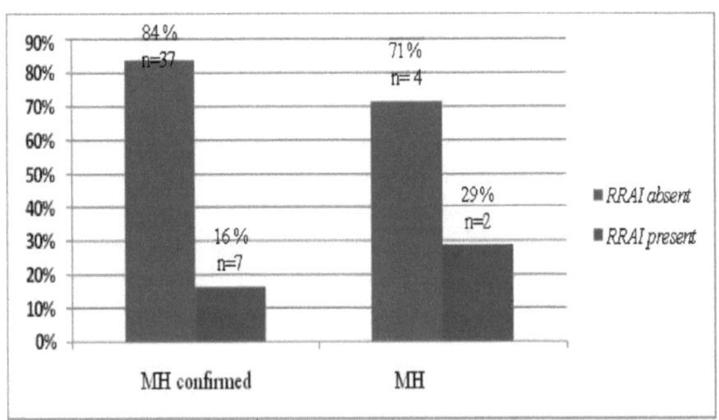

Figure 6: Results of anorectal manometry in the study population

1.5. Surgical management

Of the 69 patients with MH, 68 underwent surgery (99%). One patient was died before the operation. of the MH patients underwent surgery.

1.5.1. The operation

Endoanal Soave-type surgery was performed in 68 patients (88%). Duhamel surgery was performed in 8 patients (12%).

1.5.2. Surgical limits on the operating theatre

In the 68 operated patients, the limits of colonic resection were, to the examination definitive histopathology :

- ▶ healthy in 62 cases
- ▶ pathological in 6 cases, for the following reasons:

– An error of assessment during extemporaneous examination in one case

– Extemporaneous examination was not available in two cases, due to late surgery during the day, resulting in incomplete resection of the aganglion segment. In one patient, this incomplete resection was complicated by a perforation requiring emergency colostomy. An additional cold resection was performed in the second patient.

– A pathological proximal border on the colonic resection specimen, despite the presence of GCs in the colonic resection zone on extemporaneous and definitive examination.

– Two cases in which the surgeons not request an extemporaneous examination because of morphological evidence of a ZPT during the operation

1.6. Evolution

Of the 69 patients with MH, 53 (78%) had a good outcome, with resolution of the initial symptoms. Six deaths () occurred the study population, including one pre-operatively. These deaths were attributed to septic shock. Ten patients operated on were lost to follow-up ().

In patients without MH, the clinical course was good.

1.7. ANATOMOPATHOLOGICAL STUDY

Histopathological review of haematein-eosin slides involved 38 pre-operative surgical biopsies and 105 intra-operative biopsies taken for extemporaneous examination.

1.7.1. HISTOPATHOLOGICAL STUDY OF PRE-OPERATIVE SURGICAL BIOPSIES

Preoperative biopsies were performed in 47/80 () patients. They corresponded to :

▶ Surgical biopsies in 38 patients (81%)

▶ Superficial rectal biopsies performed with Noblett forceps in 9 patients (19%). These biopsies were taken in the private sector, which meant that they could not be re-read or included in the immunohistochemical study.

1.7.1.1. The number of cutting levels examined

The number of levels of cut per tissue block varied from 1 to 2. Two levels of cut were examined in 5/38 pre-operative biopsies (13%). An average of 1.13 levels were examined. Additional slides read for special staining (Masson's trichrome, Shiff's periodic acid and alcian blue) were not considered as cut levels (Figure 7).

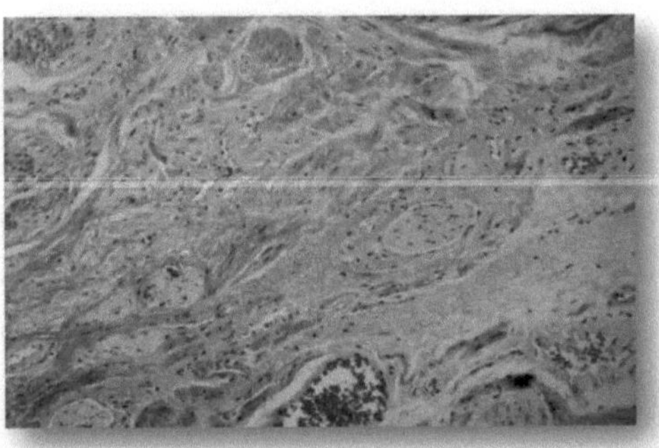

Figure 7: Histological section stained with trichrome showing hyperplastic nerve threads in a patient with Hirschsprung's disease.

1.7.1.2. Depth of pre-operative biopsies

A review of the 38 surgical biopsies showed :

▶ Twenty-nine biopsies including mucosa, submucosa and muscularis propria (76%)

- A biopsy a mucosa and sub-mucosa (3%)
- Three biopsies including submucosa and muscularis (8%)
- Four biopsies including only muscle (13%)
- A biopsy revealed only striated skeletal muscle.

1.7.1.3. Results of the rereading of slides stained with haematein-eosin

The 38 pre-operative biopsies concerned :

- MPA in 35 samples (89%)
- ZPT in 2 samples (7%)
- SPA in 1 sample (4%)

The results of the re-reading were in perfect agreement with the initial results concerning CG and nerve net hyperplasia.

1.7.1.3.1. Results rereading slides stained with haematein-eosin in areas presumed to be diseased

In patients with MH, the absence of CG and nerve hyperplasia were noted in 100% of cases (24/24 pre-operative biopsies) (Table III, Figure 8). The absence of GC was noted once, in 1/11 preoperative biopsies (9%) carried out in patients without MH (Table III). In this case, the pre-operative biopsy only involved sphincter muscle.

Table III: Results of the re-reading of haematein-eosin stained slides of pre-operative biopsies taken from presumed diseased areas

	MH confirmed (%)	MH eliminated (%)
Ganglion cells present	0	10 (91%)
Ganglion cells absent	24 (100%)	1 (9%)
Nerve nets hyperplastic	24 (100 %)	4 (36%)
Nerve nets no hyperplastic	0	7 (64%)
Total	24	11

1.7.1.3.2. Results rereading slides stained with haematein-eosin in presumed transition zones

In the two samples taken in the ZPT, GCs were absent and associated with nerve hyperplasia in both cases.

1.7.1.3.3. Results of the rereading of slides stained with haematein-eosin in areas presumed to be healthy

The sample taken in the SPA showed CGs without associated nerve hyperplasia (Figure 9).

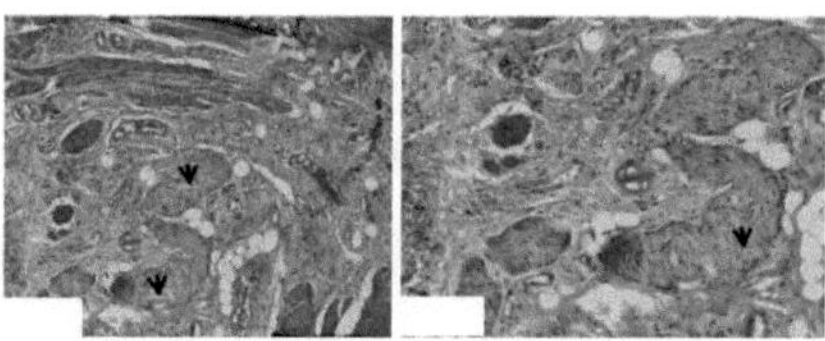

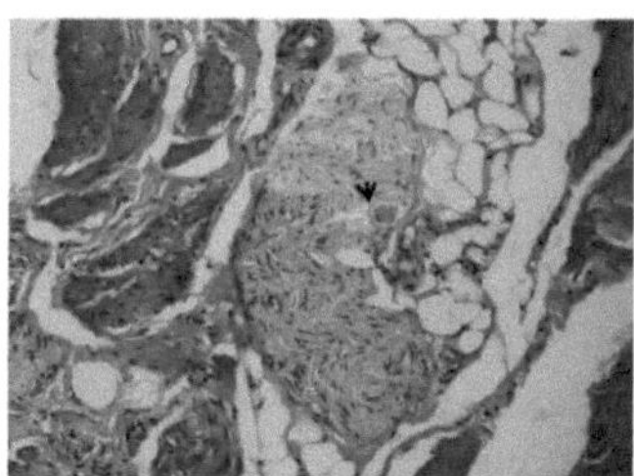

Figure 8: Histopathological examination with haematein-eosin of a pre-operative biopsy taken in an area presumed to be diseased in a patient with Hirschsprung's disease.

*(A)*Hyperplastic nerve threads (arrow)

*(B)*Hyperplastic nerve threads without ganglion cells (arrow)

Figure 9: Histopathological examination with haematein-eosin of a pre-operative biopsy taken in a presumably healthy area: presence of a lymph node cell within a nerve mesh (arrow).

1.7.2. Histopathological study of intraoperative samples

Intraoperative sampling for extemporaneous examination was performed in 52/69 patients with HD (75%). Only one patient without HD underwent extemporaneous examination.

1.7.2.1. Different areas of intraoperative biopsies analysed extemporaneously

A total of 105 biopsies were sent for extemporaneous examination from 53 patients, only one of whom was free of MH. Multiple samples from different areas were taken in some cases for the same patient. The distribution of areas was as follows:

- ▶ 48 biopsies carried out in the SPA (46%)
- ▶ 22 biopsies performed in the ZPT (21%)

▶ 35 biopsies performed in the MPA (33%)

1.7.2.2. The different parietal layers of intraoperative biopsies :

The various biopsies performed were panparietal in 92 cases (88%), irrespective of the area biopsied (Table IV).

Table IV: The different parietal layers of intraoperative biopsies

Wall layers	Number	Frequency
Mucous membrane,	92	88 %
submucosa and muscularis		
Mucosa and sub-mucosa	3	2 %
Muscular	10	10 %
Total	105	100 %

1.7.2.3. Histopathological study of intraoperative biopsies

Extemporaneous examination of the biopsies confirmed the diagnosis of MH by the absence of CG in 34 out of 35 biopsies in the MPA (97%). The nerve threads were hyperplastic in 27/35 cases (79%) in the MPA (Figures 10 and 11). CG and nerve hyperplasia were observed in 15/22 biopsies (68%) and 13/22 biopsies (59%) taken in ZPT respectively (Figure 10 and 11).CG and nerve hyperplasia were observed respectively in 47/48 biopsies (97%) and in 5/48 biopsies (10%) taken in SPAs (Figure 10 and 11). Biopsy of the MH-free patient showed CGs without associated nerve hyperplasia. The results of the review were in perfect agreement with the final results for identification of GCs. Discordance in the assessment of nerve net hyperplasia was observed in 7 cases (7%).

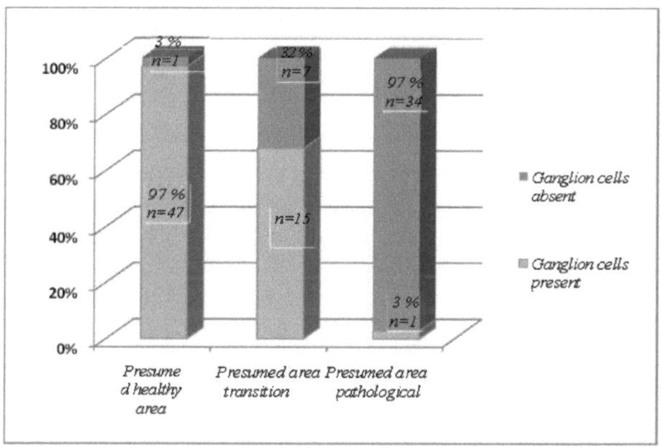

Figure 10: Distribution of lymph node cells in intraoperative biopsies according to area

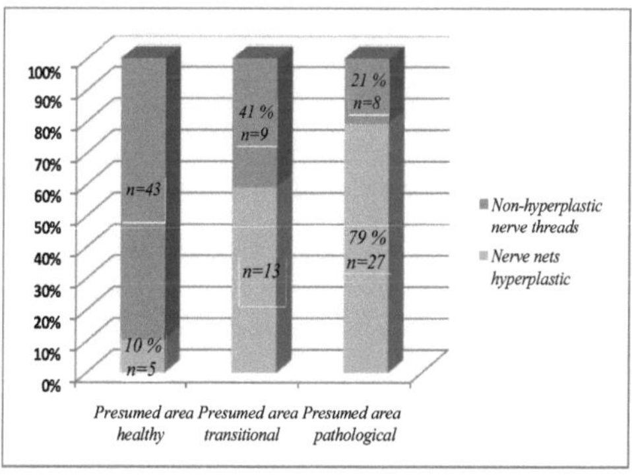

Figure 11: Nerve net hyperplasia in intraoperative biopsies according to area

1.7.2.4. Concordance between the result of extemporaneous examination and the result of the the final examination

The results of the extemporaneous and definitive examinations were :

▶ Concordant in 51 cases (98%)

▶ Discordant in 1 case (1%)

▶ The response was delayed in one case (1%) when an extemporaneous biopsy was performed on an appendectomy specimen, despite the absence of CG

The discrepancy observed concerned a patient with trisomy 21 operated on at the age of 8, whose extemporaneous examination had revealed GCs not found during the definitive examination.

1.8. STUDY IMMUNOHISTOCHEMISTRY WITH ANTICOPRS ANTI-CALRETININ

The immunohistochemical study with the anti-calretinin antibody involved 110 biopsies. belonging to 68 patients, including 60 with MH.

1.8.1. CALRETININ EXPRESSION IN BIOPSIES FROM PATIENTS WITH HIRSCHSPRUNG'S DISEASE

In the 60 patients with MH:

▶ 45 biopsies were taken from the MPA, 4 of which contained no chorion, muscularis mucosae or submucosa

▶ 16 biopsies concerned the ZPT

▶ 40 biopsies were taken from the SPA, 6 of which had no mucosa or muscularis mucosa

1.8.1.1. Expression of calretinin in biopsies taken presumed diseased areas

In patients with HD, calretinin confirmed the absence of CG in 43/45 ZPM biopsies (96%). It also confirmed the absence of interstitial nerve fibres in 38/41 MPA biopsies (93%).

Calretinin showed the presence of CG in 2/45 MPA biopsies (4%). Interstitial nerve fibres were labelled in 3 of 41 MPA specimens (7%) (Tables VI, VII). The expression of interstitial nerve fibres and CGs were concomitant except in one case.

1.8.1.2. Expression of calretinin in biopsies taken presumed transition zones

Samples taken from the ZPT showed interstitial nerve fibre and CG markers in 10 of 16 biopsies (63%) (Tables VI and VII).

1.8.1.3. Expression of calretinin in biopsies taken from presumed healthy areas

Labelling with the anti-calretinin antibody resulted in brown labelling of GCs. This was cytoplasmic and nuclear (Figure 12). Granular marking of the nerve threads was constantly associated (Figure 13).

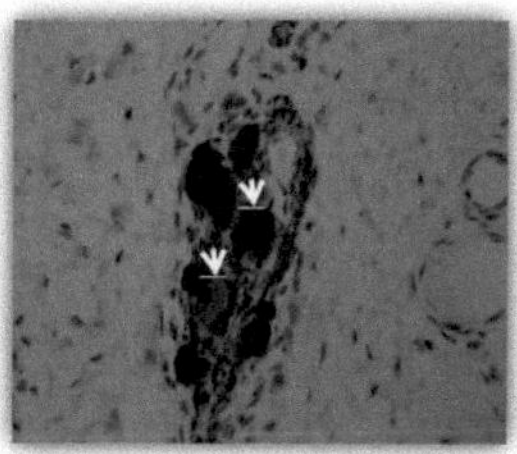
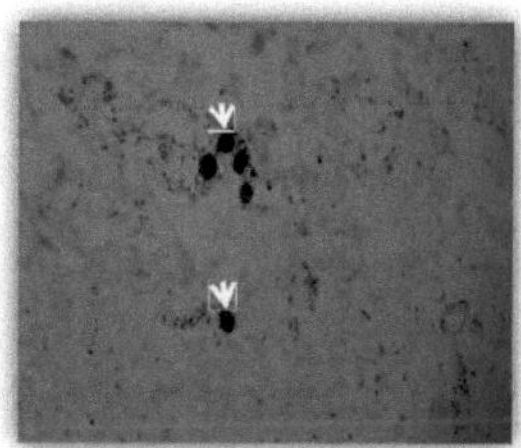

Figure 12: Anti-calretinin antibody labelling of lymph node cells in a biopsy taken from a presumably healthy area in a patient with Hirschsprung's disease.

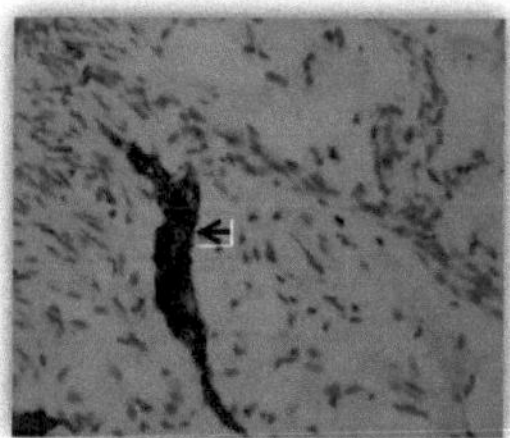
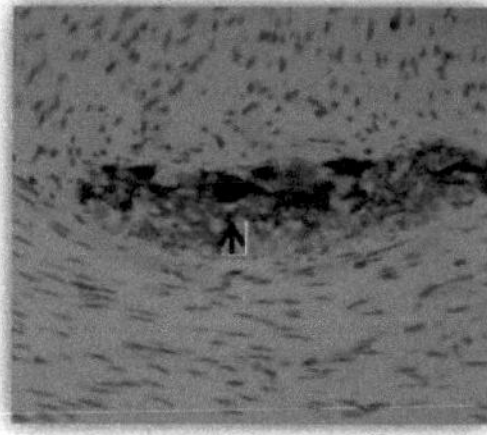

Figure 13: Anti-calretinin antibody labelling of nerve threads in a biopsy taken from a presumably healthy area in a patient with Hirschsprung's disease.

Granular marking of interstitial nerve fibres was observed in the chorion, muscularis mucosa and submucosa of biopsies taken in the SPA (Figure 14).

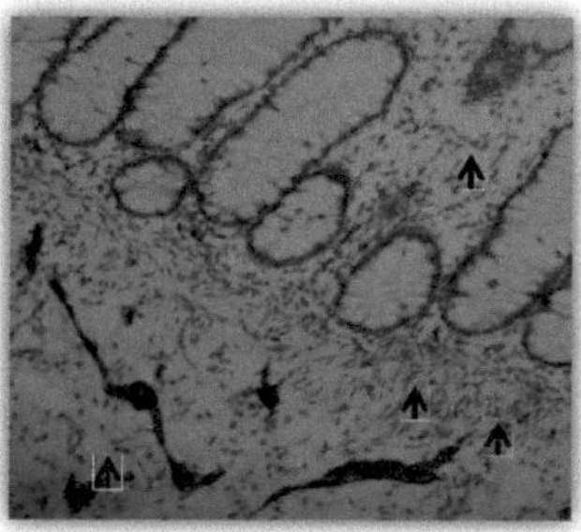

Figure 14: Labelling of interstitial nerve fibres by the anti-calretinin antibody (arrowhead) in the chorion, muscularis mucosae and submucosae on a biopsy from a presumably healthy area in a patient with Hirschsprung's disease.

The results of the immunohitochemical study on biopsies taken in SPAs showed (Tables V and VI):

▶ Labelled GCs in 35 biopsies out of 40 (88%)

▶ Interstitial nerve fibres were labelled in the different parietal layers in 31 of 34 biopsies (91%). Marking was more frequent in the chorion and muscularis mucosae (91%) than in the submucosa (87%) (Tables V and VI).

▶ Nerve net markings were present in all cases

Table V: Zonal expression of calretinin by ganglion cells and interstitial nerve fibres in patients with Hirschsprung's disease

Histological parameters	Biopsy area		
	ZPM N (%)	ZPT N (%)	SPA N (%)
Cells	2/45	10/16	35/40
lymph node	(4 %)	(63 %)	(88 %)
Nerve fibres	3/41	10/16	31/34
interstitial	(7 %)	(63 %)	(91 %)

Table VI: Expression of calretinin by interstitial nerve fibres in the different parietal layers, depending on the area, in patients with Hirschsprung's disease.

Nerve fibres ZPM ZPT ZPS		
interstitial N (%)	N (%)	N (%)
3/41	10/16	31/34*
(7 %)	(63 %)	(91 %)
Muscular 3/41	10/16	31/34**
mucosa (7 %)	(63 %)	(91 %)
Chorion 3/41	10/16	32/37***
Submucosa (7 %)	(63 %)	(87 %)

(*) 6 mucosa-free biopsies

(**) 6 biopsies without muscular mucosa (***) 3 biopsies without submucosa

1.8.2. Calretinin expression in biopsies from patients without Hirschsprung's disease:

MH was eliminated in 8 patients. The nine biopsies taken from these patients were divided into the following zones:

▶ Eight MPA biopsies

▶ A biopsy in an SPA

In the MPAcalretinin expression resulted in :

▶ Concomitant labelling of CGs and interstitial nerve fibres in 7 cases. This labelling was identical to that observed on biopsies taken in ZPS in patients with MH

▶ The absence of labelling of CGs and interstitial nerve fibres in one case was consistent the result histopathological examination with haematein-eosin, but inconsistent with the final clinical diagnosis. The biopsy in question included only sphincter striated muscles. The diagnosis of MH in this patient was overturned in view of the good clinical course.

The only case in the SPA showed expression of calretinin by both CGs and interstitial nerve fibres.

2. Analytical study of the diagnostic performance of the immunohistochemical study using the anti-calretinin antibody

The analytical study covered the 53 samples taken in the MPA. These samples belonged to 46 patients with HD and 7 patients without the disease. Comparison of the diagnosis made on the basis of the immunohistochemical study with the anti-calretinin antibody and that obtained on histopathological examination of the haematein-eosin stained slides showed that calretinin correctly confirmed the diagnosis of MH in 43/46 patients with the disease and correctly invalidated it in all patients without the disease (Table VII).

Table VII: Analysis of concordance between immunohistochemical diagnosis with anti-calretinin antibody and histopathological diagnosis with haematein-eosin

		Diagnosis			
		MH* confirmed	MH*eliminated		
Immunohistochemical diagnosis		histopathological examination with haematein-eosin	histopathological examination with haematein-eosin	Total	K
Calretinin	Negative test	43	0	43	0,791
	Positive test	3	7	10	
	Total	46	7	53	

MH*= Hirschsprung's disease.

The sensitivity, specificity, positive predictive value and negative predictive value of the anti-calretinin antibody in the diagnosis of MH were 93%, 100%, 100%, and 70% respectively. The agreement between the results of the immunohistochemical study with the anti-calretinin antibody and the result of the histopathological study with haematene eosin was good, with a coefficient K=0.791 (Table VIII).

Table VIII: Diagnostic performance of calretinin in the diagnosis of Hirschsprung's disease

	Se*(%)	Sp**(%)	PPV***(%)	VPN****(%)	K
Calretinin	93%	100 %	100%	70%	0,791

Se*= sensitivity; Sp**= specificity; PPV***: positive predictive value; NPV:**** negative predictive value

Three false negatives were observed. They involved two newborns aged 3 and 5 days and a 2-year-old infant. All biopsies were pre-operative biopsies and therefore had not undergone anterior cryofixation. Labelling with the anti-calretinin antibody showed the concomitant presence of CG and interstitial nerve fibres in two cases. Calretinin positivity in the 3rd case was based on interstitial nerve fibre positivity alone. The 3 patients underwent surgery for a rectal, sigmoidianal and left colonic form. The clinical course was good in all 3 cases, with resolution of the symptomatology. after resection of the diseased colonic segment. false positives were observed based on the results of the histopathological examination. haematein and eosin.

DISCUSSION

Our study included a total of 80 patients, 69 of whom had MH. Anti-calretinin antibody labelling of biopsies taken in the presumed healthy zone (PHZ) resulted in chromogenic nuclear and cytoplasmic deposition of GCs and granular deposition in interstitial nerve fibres. This was identical to that observed in biopsies taken from presumed diseased areas (PDAs) in patients without HD. In SPZs, interstitial nerve fibres expressed calretinin more frequently (91%) than CGs (89%). Anti-calretinin antibody labelled CGs and interstitial nerve fibres in 63% of biopsies taken in ZPT. In the MPA biopsies, CGs were labelled in 2 biopsies, while interstitial nerve fibres were labelled in 3 biopsies (7.3%), resulting in 3 false negatives. No false positives were observed. The sensitivity, specificity, positive predictive value and negative predictive value of the anti-calretinin antibody were 93%, 100%, 100% and 70% respectively, with good agreement (k=0.791).

1. Pathophysiology

The gastrointestinal system is distinguished from other systems by the richness of its innervation. It has two types of innervation: extrinsic innervation represented essentially by the parasympathetic autonomic nervous system, and intrinsic innervation capable of autonomic function independent of the extrinsic system [17].

The enteric nervous system is made up of :

- The meyenteric plexus, which lies between the two muscular layers controls motricity
- The submucosal plexus, located between the muscularis and the intestinal mucosa, which coordinates digestive secretions.
- Interstitial nerve fibres in the chorion, which make up Isawa's mucosal plexus, the role of which remains unknown [18]

In HD, there is a disruption of the migration and differentiation process of neural crest cells in the enteral nervous system, governed by the RET gene.
"Rearranged during transfection (RET) and its ligands. This disruption leads to a total absence of CG in the various plexuses, leading to overactivity of the intestine with permanent release acetylcholine. This leads to continuous contraction of the affected colonic segment and progressive secondary dilatation of the healthy overlying colon [3,19].

The involvement interstitial nerve fibres in the genesis of HD is not clearly elucidated. Indeed, no study explains the absence of interstitial nerve fibres in aganglionic segments [10,12-15]. Other studies report disruption of inhibitory neurotransmitters that relax intestinal smooth muscle, such as vasoactive intestinal peptide, substance P, enkephalins and nitric oxide [19].

2. Genetic study

HD a congenital disease, most often sporadic, with only 5-20% of cases in families. Its transmission is complex, involving multigene involvement. Penetrance is low, variable and sex-dependent. It is twice as common in boys as in girls. Its onset often involves multigene involvement. The main gene involved is the RET proto-oncogene [1]. It is located on the long arm of chromosome 10 (10q11.2) and comprises 21 exons. It found in around 35% of sporadic cases and 49% of familial cases[1,20] . Damage to the RET gene is frequently associated with long forms MH. The RET gene codes for a 114 amino acid transmembrane receptor with an extracellular cadherin-like domain and an intracellular tyrosine kinase domain. It is responsible for proliferation, differentiation and migration of neural crest cells [17].

Mutation of this gene has been implicated in the genesis of HD as well as in the appearance of type 2 multiple neuroendocrine neoplasia. Mutations in the RET gene that lead HD can affect any coding part of the gene's 21 exons, and more 100 different mutations have been identified. Some of the haplotypes formed act as protective factors, while others predispose to HD or help to determine its extent. The polymorphism of the mutations identified and the exons involved, on the one , and the variable penetrance of the RET gene, on the other, make it difficult to carry out an antenatal diagnosis or molecular diagnosis of HD [1].

RET mutations are also associated with severe and complicated forms (stoma, episode of enterocolitis, double operation). In a retrospective study of 42 cases of HD by Ramos et al, the RET mutation was observed in 53.3% of severe forms compared with only 15.3% of so-called mild forms, with no significant difference between two groups [20]. These so-called severe forms could therefore be an indication for testing for the mutation. Other genes involved in HD are only identified in 5 to 10% of cases. They correspond essentially to ligands of the RET receptor: glial-derived neurotrophic factor, endothelin 3 and B, the SOX10 transcription factor and the PHOX2B gene [1]. Unlike RET mutations in HD, mutations in multiple neurendocrine neoplasia type 2 are activating mutations. As a result, the association of these two diseases in the same families and in the same patients is unlikely. Although rare, it has been observed in 2.5% of patients [20]. This unlikely association could be the result of molecular mechanisms occurring at different periods of embryonic and postnatal life [1]. In our series, there were two familial cases. The genetic study could not be due to a lack of technical resources.

3. Epidemiological study

3.1. Breakdown of patients by gender

In our study, the majority of patients with HD were male, with a sex ratio (boy/girl) of 3.6. This male predominance has been found in several studies with a sex ratio between 3 and 4 (Table IX) [5,21,22].

Table IX: Breakdown patients with Hirschsprung's disease by sex

Study	Male sex	Female sex	Sex ratio
Menezes 2006 [23] (259 cases)	200 (77,2%)	59 (22,8%)	3,32
Swenson 1973 [22] (501 cases)	406 (81%)	95 (19%)	4,3
Ikeda [21] (1628 cases)	1220 (75%)	408 (25%)	3
Our study	54 (78%)	15 (22%)	3,6

The study carried out at the regional paediatric surgery centre in Monastir found this to be the case.male preponderance, with a sex ratio of 4 [5]. The inversion of the sex ratio in total and extensive colonic forms has been observed in the literature [9,24]. In our series, two of the 3 extensive forms were observed in girls.

3.2. Breakdown of patients age

MH is a congenital disease whose clinical onset is most often neonatal. Diagnosis is made in 65% of cases before the age of 1 month and in 95% of cases before the age of one year [25].

The same is true in our study, where 80% of patients were diagnosed at neonatal age, and 99% at less than 2 years of age. Only one case was discovered late, at the age of 15. Our results were similar to those described by Ikeda [21], where 48.7% of cases were discovered in the first month of life and 83.4% by the end of the first year. The discovery of HD children is less frequent, with a peak in frequency at the in 2-year-old age group [5]. It is exceptional adults and usually affects young adults with ranging from 16 to 74 years of age [26].

4. CLINICAL STUDY

4.1. FORMS OF HIRSCHSPRUNG'S DISEASE

In HD, the lower limit of the extent of the pathological zone is always the internal anal sphincter, while the upper limit varies in height and determines the different forms of this disease. Depending on the extent of the aganglionosis [5] :

- The short or "classic" form, involving rectal and recto-sigmoid forms (88% of cases)

- The long form extends to the left, transverse and right colon and the pancolic form (8 to 10% of cases).

- Total colonic form extending into the small intestine (1% of cases)

The classic recto-sigmoid form accounted for 83% of cases in our series. This form accounted for 80% of Ikeda's series [21]. The presence of a discontinuous form of MH has been reported in the literature, where aganglionic zones alternate with zones containing CG. This form of MH is rare and could explain the presence of a pathological border on an endoanal resection specimen in a patient whose extemporaneous and definitive intraoperative biopsy results showed the presence of CGs [7,27].

4.2. FAMILY HISTORY AND CONSANGUINITY

Most cases of HD are sporadic. Familial forms HD vary from 5 to 20% [28,29]. In our series, a family history of HD was reported in only one case. In the Tunisian study by Fkih, familial cases accounted for 9.5% [5]. The frequency of family history correlates with the extent of the disease. The frequency of familial forms rises from 3.2% in long forms to 11.3% in total forms [21]. Consanguinity, on the other hand, has been little studied in the various studies of HD [1,25].

4.3. THE SIGNSCLINICAL OF DISCOVERY OF THE DISEASE HIRSCHSPRUNG'S DISEASE

4.3.1. THE MECONIUM EMISSION DELAY

In the physiological state, meconium is emitted during the first 48 hours of life. Delayed meconium emission of more than 48 hours was observed in 70% of cases in our study. This clinical sign often reveals HD and is observed in 40.6 to 58% of patients [21].

Delayed meconium emission in HD has a sensitivity of 83%, a specificity of 88% and a positive predictive value of 77% for newborns suspected having HD [5,21]. This sign is also observed in cases of prematurity, small bowel atresia, meconium ileus, dehydration, anal stenosis, imperforate anus and anal or rectal agenesis [5].

4.3.2. INTESTINAL OBSTRUCTION

HD is the most common cause of lower intestinal obstruction in neonates. It accounts for 1/3 of all causes of neonatal obstruction [5]. Other causes of neonatal obstruction should be investigated, such as meconium ileus and left small bowel syndrome [21]. In our seriesintestinal obstruction was found in 71% of cases (49/69 patients). with HD). This clinical sign has a sensitivity of 86% and a specificity of 13% [5].

4.3.3. CHRONIC CONSTIPATION :

Chronic constipation is a frequently revealing sign of HD. Its appearance from birth should strongly suggest HD [5,19]. It is more frequent in infants and children aged over 2 years, where it is observed in 68.7% to 79.3% of cases [19]. This sign was observed in 44% of our patients with HD. This could be explained by the predominance of neonates in our study population.

5. RADIOLOGICAL AND FUNCTIONAL INVESTIGATIONS :

5.1. THE OPAQUE ENEMA

An opaque enema is the first test to be carried out when HD is suspected. It is used to locate the PTZ and to guide the surgical approach to the patient [5,6]. The interpretation of the opaque enema is based on the search for signs colonic distension and stricture, abnormalities of the colonic wall suggestive of enterocolitis and a zone of disparity in calibre or "ZPT". This zone is the most specific sign of HD and is observed radiologically in the form of an inverted cone. Pathophysiologically, it reflects the disparity in calibre between the dilated ganglion segment and the narrowed aganglion segment [5]. In our study, ZPT was detected in 43/63 (68%) of the enemas performed in patients with HD. The sensitivity of the opaque enema in identifying the ZPT varies from 68 to 94% of cases of HD, and is lower in neonates and in extensive forms [5]. False negatives are associated with rectal touching or evacuating enemas prior to radiological examination [29]. Bone landmarks can be used to identify the site of the ZPT and thus assess the extent of the MH [5]. The concordance rate between histological and radiological ZPT varies from 63-90% [5]. Short forms HD also difficult to diagnose radiologically and require direct insertion of the rectal probe just above the anal canal [5,6].

5.2. Anorectal manometry

Anorectal manometry is a dynamic test which assesses the response of the internal sphincter to distension of the rectal ampulla by studying the pressures along the anal canal [5,21]. The reliability of this test becomes excellent 12 days after birth when the recto-enteric reflex becomes normal [5].In HD, rectal distension does not cause any relaxation of the internal sphincter, revealing hypertonia. The absence of this reflex is highly suggestive of HD but remains non-specific as it is observed in achalasia of the anal canal, in chronic constipated patients with megacolon and in patients less than 3 weeks old [28]. In our series, the recto-anal reflex was absent in 37/44 (84%) patients with HD. The sensitivity of anorectal manometry varies in the literature from 70 to 93% [5,21].

6. Therapeutic management: The surgical procedure

HD is treated surgically. The diseased area is resected and digestive continuity is re-established during the same operation. Different techniques are proposed depending on the experience of the team:

▶ The Swenson procedure, which involves performing a direct colo-anal anastomosis [5].
▶ The Duhamel procedure, which consists of keeping the diseased rectum with a healthy colon lowered into the posterior sacral concavity [28].
▶ The Soave procedure is a surgical technique which involves lowering the healthy colon into the rectum, the mucosa of which has been resected. Preservation of the rectal wall minimises the risk of nerve damage in the pelvis [28].

In our study, 88% of patients underwent Soave surgery and 12% Duhamel surgery. The Soave technique is currently the most widely used, particularly for short forms of MH.

7. EVOLUTION

The outcome was good in 77% of patients. The five immediate postoperative deaths were attributed to septic shock. In Ikeda's series, which included 1,628 patients with HD, 115 deaths were recorded. Septic shock was also the most frequent cause of death (40.9%) [21].

8. ANATOMOPATHOLOGICAL STUDY

8.1. THE DIFFERENT TYPES OF PRE-OPERATIVE BIOPSY

8.1.1. SUPERFICIAL RECTAL BIOPSIES USING NOBLETT FORCEPS

Superficial rectal biopsy with Noblett forceps is an aspiration biopsy that does not require general anaesthesia or sutures. It is performed by a catheter inserted into the rectum, which removes a small fragment of the colonic wall via a vacuum created at its tip. This fragment comprises a submucosa, a muscular mucosa and a mucosa [30].Complications are exceptional. In a series of 1,000 pre-operative biopsies carried out by Quinn et al, the rate of severe rectal bleeding and rectal perforation exceed 0.2% [13]. In many referral centres, superficial rectal biopsy has completely replaced surgical biopsy as the diagnostic method. It has level C diagnostic evidence in the taxonomy of recommendations [30].However, the small size of some biopsies is responsible for 6-9% of inconclusive results[31], which are more frequent in children aged over 5 years [7,12,13,30]. This is explained by oedema of the mucosa and an increase in fibrous tissue, which make it difficult to take adequate samples from the submucosa [31].

In a systematic review of the literature including 22 articles, superficial rectal biopsies showed a better diagnostic performance than radiological and endoscopic explorations with an average sensitivity of 93% and an average specificity of 98% (confidence interval=95%) [32]. The diagnostic accuracy of superficial rectal biopsies was found to be better in infants (100%) than in neonates (90%) [33]. To reduce the rate of inconclusive results linked to inadequate biopsies (Figure 17), the 2009 International Gastroenterology Committee defined criteria for evaluating pre-operative biopsies, which are necessary to ensure correct interpretation [13]:

At least two biopsies should be required, with a minimum diameter of 3mm. Biopsies should include as much mucosa as submucosa. The biopsy should be well oriented and included in the correct axis avoid loss of tissue between the different levels of tissue block section. Pre-operative biopsies should be taken at least 2 cm above the pectineal line. This area is physiologically devoid of CG and shows hyperplasia of the nerve nets.The International Gastroenterology Committee even recommends that biopsies be taken at different levels, i.e. 2, 3 and 5 cm above the pectineal line, to avoid missing short forms of HD [13].

The presence of striated skeletal muscle, transitional epithelium or squamous epithelium means that the biopsy is inadequate. However, the presence of even a single GC in this area formally rules out HD and a 2nd biopsy is not necessary in this case [11].

In our series, one of the surgical biopsies was inadequate because of its low location. The histopathological diagnosis concluded that there was no GC, in contradiction with the clinical course, which ruled out the diagnosis of HD. In the majority of studies, superficial preoperative biopsies lacking submucosa were among the main causes of biopsies (76.5%), followed by distal biopsies (17.6%) [11,13].

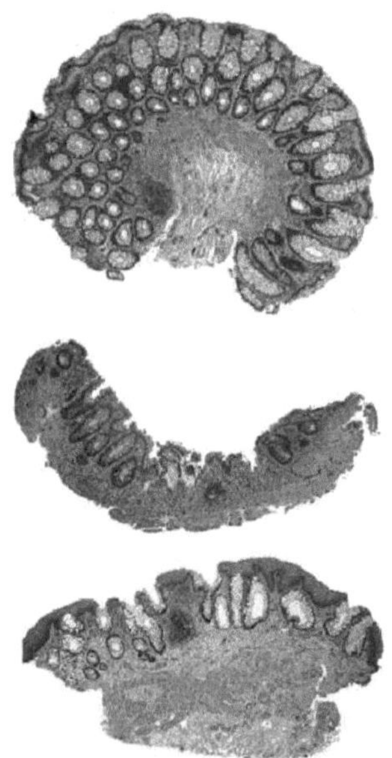

Adequate biopsy 2-3 mm long, more than 1/3 of which is sub-mucosa

Inadequate biopsy due to sub-mucosal defect

Biopsy inadequate by presence squamous anal mucosa

Figure 15: Examples of superficial rectal biopsies [13].

8.1.2. SURGICAL BIOPSIES

All preoperative biopsies in our series were surgical, performed under general anaesthesia [13]. This was the most commonly used method, as the Noblett forceps were not available in the paediatric surgery department at Habib Thameur Hospital. Surgical biopsies are associated with an increased risk of complications, which increases with the depth of the biopsy [13]. Complications include rectal discharge, infection and perforation [30]. They are indicated immediately in children from the age of 4 or after inadequate or inconclusive Noblett forceps biopsies [31].Surgical biopsies may be limited the muscularis and subserosa or include the entire thickness of the wall. The advantage of surgical biopsies is that they can confirm or rule out muscle involvement and include Auerbach's plexuses, which richer in GCs [7,13]. In our series, 76% and 89% of the preoperative and extemporaneous biopsies included all of the muscles. the colonic wall and 10% and 13% of them were limited to the muscularis. Although these biopsies were surgical, 3% of them included the mucosa and submucosa. This may be due to a problem with the orientation of the biopsy fragment when it was embedded in paraffin, resulting in tissue loss during sectioning [9].

8.2. ENZYME-LINKED IMMUNOSORBENT ASSAY USING ACETYLCHOLINESTERASE

The acetylcholinesterase study is an enzyme-linked immunosorbent assay used to label extrinsic nerve nets in the enteric nervous system [7]. Together with histological examination of slides stained with haematein-eosin, it is the reference method diagnosing MH in several centres [7]. It is performed on fresh frozen tissue and on 15 µm thick sections. It therefore requires an additional biopsy in addition to the one dedicated to histological examination haematein-eosin. Interpretation requires the simultaneous presence of a positive control and a negative control [7]. Extrinsic innervation is accentuated in patients with HD. Extrinsic nerve fibres are increased in density and thickness in the chorion, muscularis mucosae and submucosa in diseased areas (Figure 18). The hyper-reactivity of the nerve nets to acetylcholinesterase observed in the muscularis mucosae is pathognomonic of HD, whereas that of the chorion can be observed during intestinal neuronal dysplasia [18]. The positivity of the acetylcholinesterase enzyme-linked immunosorbent assay is variable and results in lower density acetylcholinesterase-positive fibres, giving rise false negatives [9]. This is explained by some authors by a different and physiologically less important parasympathetic innervation of the transverse and ascending colonic segment [34]. False positives in the acetylcholinesterase enzyme-linked immunosorbent assay are extremely rare. Most studies report a specificity of 100% [35]. False positives are explained by extravasation of acetylcholinesterase from red blood cells during haemorrhagic biopsies [34].The false negative rate varies from 0 to 40%. Its sensitivity varies between 85% and 93.5% [14,35]. False negatives are associated with superficial biopsies that do not include muscularis mucosae, and with the immaturity of the enzyme system in children under 2 months of age [13]. This method is not currently available in our department, as it is time-consuming, takes 90 minutes to perform, requires the use of toxic products and has a short validity period. In addition, the difficulty of interpreting the labelling, inter-observer discordance and the variability of cholinergic innervation in premature babies and in extensive forms HD are all obstacles to the use of the acetylcholinesterase enzyme-linked immunosorbent assay [36-38].

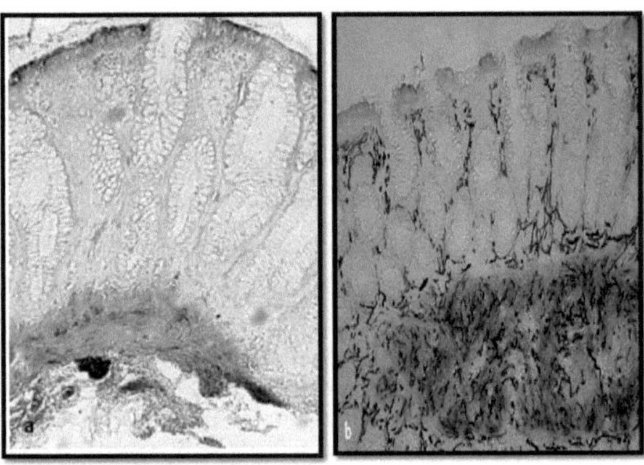

Figure 16: Acetylcholinesterase enzyme-linked immunosorbent assay

A: Result of the acetylcholinesterase enzyme-linked immunosorbent assay in a subject without Hirschsrpung's disease: absence of extrinsic nerve fibre hyperplasia.

B: Extrinsic nerve fibres of increased density, labelled by acetylcholinesterase in the chorion, muscularis mucosae and submucosa of a patient with Hirschsprung's disease [1].

8.3. Histopathological study of hematein-stained slides Eosin :

Histological examination of slides stained with haematein-eosin with or without a study of acetylcholinesterase enzyme-linked immunosorbent assay is the reference method for diagnosing MH. It is still the most commonly used method [1,13,34,39]. The diagnostic performance of haematein is variable from one study to another. It is thought to depend essentially on the number levels of section taken. , Kapur et al. assert that the rate of discordance in haematein-eosin can be avoided by using a large number of sections [7]. The diagnostic performance of the haematein-eosin study varies between 78.3% and 95% [13,16,39]. Other authors report lower specificity and sensitivity (37.7% and 54.4%). However, the number of levels performed was not specified in these studies [35]. Combining the haematein-eosin test with a study of the immuno-enzymatic activity of acetylcholinesterase or an immunohistochemical study increases its diagnostic performance to 99.7% [34].

8.3.1. Number of levels of tissue cutting recommended :

In our study, 2 slice levels were read in 13% of cases.Current standard practice for the examination of biopsies taken for suspected neuromuscular disorders of the enteric system is the subject of numerous discrepancies, in particular concerning the number of levels of section to be performed before a diagnosis of MH can be made [13]. Of the 86 European and American pathology centres that manage this type of biopsy, only 33 perform more than one level of section. In these centres, the number of levels performed varies from 15 to 75 depending on the author [13]. To limit these discrepancies, the most recent International Gastroenterology Committee recommends that 50 to 75 levels of section be performed and read for an initial examination, and that other levels be repeated if no GC is identified [12,13,40]. In other centres, cut levels may be performed until all the blocks have used up, as long as no GCs are observed [41]. This makes histological diagnosis of MH using haematein-eosin a fastidious, restrictive and time-consuming procedure. The number of levels is a decisive factor in the correct diagnosis of HD. In the study by Serafini et al., 54. of GCs were found level 50 [16], and In another study, 24.5% of biopsies re-examined on different levels showed the appearance of GCs initially absent on the first levels produced [40].In our study, despite the common practice of a single cutting level, no unnecessary operations were reported. However, additional slides were taken for special staining (Masson's Trichrome, Shiff's Periodic Acid and Alcian Blue). Special stains can be used to rule out other differential diagnoses such as congenital or acquired fibrotic disorders seen in certain myopathies [7].

8.3.2. Histopathological study of hematein and eosin slides of biopsies taken from healthy areas:

GCs are large cells measuring between 25 and 40 µm. They are recognised on histological examination as cells with abundant eosinophilic cytoplasm and an eccentric nucleus with a prominent eosinophilic nucleolus (Figure 19 A). These cells are best identified in the meyenteric plexus, where they are more numerous [42]. They are less numerous in children aged over 2 years [31]. They are more difficult to identify in neonates because the GCs are immature, with less cytoplasm, a hyperchromatic nucleus and a less prominent nucleolus (Figure 17 B) [36]. They may therefore be confused with fibroblasts, endothelial cells or plasma cells, resulting in false negatives [16,39]. The immaturity of neonatal GCs is difficult to assess and few pathologists give an opinion on the maturity of GCs, even in specialist paediatric centres [43]. Enzyme-linked immunosorbent assay using succinate dehydrogenase is the only objective means of identifying GC maturity. In our study, 79% of our population were neonates. CG identification was nevertheless easy, with mature-looking CGs. CG immaturity at birth is physiological [43]. Maturation occurs progressively from the first weeks of life until three months after birth, which may explain the mature appearance of GCs in the majority of our population [44]. Assessment of the presence or absence of GCs is the main histological criterion in the diagnosis of HD.

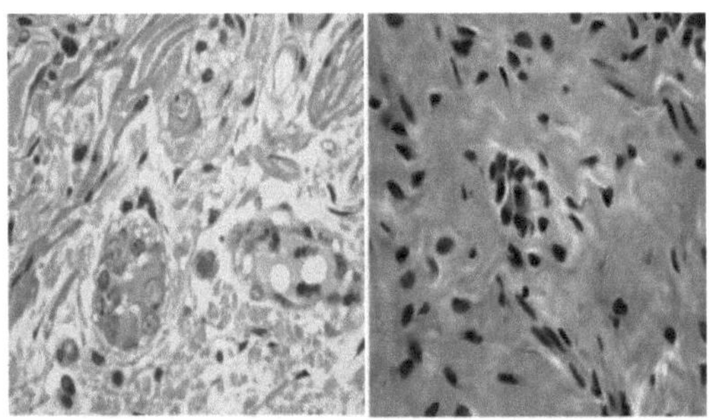

Figure 17: Haematein-eosin stained sections showing A: Mature lymph node cells B: Immature ganglion cells with hyperchromatic nuclei and sparse cytoplamse [43].

8.3.3. HISTOLOGICAL STUDY OF HEMATEIN AND EOSIN SLIDES OF BIOPSIES TAKEN IN THE TRANSITION ZONE

The extent of the transition zone is difficult to estimate, although several authors agree that it is limited to the 3-5cm following the diseased area. Its length depends on several factors, including the extent of the MH[45]. It is vital to identify the transition zone. The persistence of a transition zone the unresected colon is associated with persistent and sometimes severe colonic motor disorders. In a meta-analysis by Friedmacher et al, which included 29 articles over a period of 26 years, the persistence of colonic motor disorders after resection in the diseased zone or transition zone was reported in 34.4% of cases [46]. The transition zone is reflected histologically by the appearance of CGs and the persistence of extrinsic nerve net hyperplasia [47]. In our study, GCs were present in 68% of biopsies (15/22) and nerve net hyperplasia was observed in 59% of specimens (13/22). The retrospective nature of our study and the small number of specimens taken in the transition zone were obstacles to the interpretation of these results.

8.3.3.1. Ganglion cells

The presence of GCs marks the beginning of the transition zone and the end of the diseased zone. The appearance of GCs in Auerbach's and Meissner's plexuses is generally concomitant. However, some authors report the first appearance of GCs in Auerbach's plexus [47].

Several studies [47-49] use the reduced number of GCs as the main criterion for identifying the transition zone. This criterion is rarely applied, due to the lack of reliable practical values for establishing a normal density of GCs. Moreover, the various published values are very inconsistent [47]. In order to gain a better understanding of the mode of appearance of GCs in the transition zone, several authors [45,47,48] have taken colonic samples, included in their entirety, around their entire circumference, along the entire length of the transtion zone. Reading whole section slices showed that the reappearance of GCs was progressive and heterogeneous. In fact, GCs were not found around the entire circumference of a transition zone: ganglionic areas alternated with aganglionic areas in at least 1/8 of the colonic circumference, in both Auerbach's and Meissner's plexuses (Figure 18) [50]. This heterogeneous distribution of GCs is explained by longitudinal rather than transverse caudal extension of the GCs [50]. This implies the need to examine circumferential sections during extemporaneous examinations to correctly identify the transition zone. Moreover, extemporaneous examination is performed on circumferential colonic biopsies in many reference centres [45,48,50]. In addition to the reduced number of GCs, some authors [45,50] have identified isolated GCs in the muscularis layer or in the subserosal layer, not connected to the nerve bundles, as well as ectopic GCs in the subserosal layer in the transition zone. These 2 criteria were found in 56 out of 59 samples by Kapur et al. and could explain the functional alteration of the GCs in the transition zone [47].

8.3.3.2. Nerve hyperplasia

Nerve hyperplasia is a criterion for identifying both the diseased area and the transition zone. However, it is inconstant the transition zone [50]. This the case in our study, where nerve hyperplasia was observed in 59% of samples from the transition zone. This hyperplasia concerns extrinsic nerve threads which can be identified by the presence of intra-neuronal collagen and perineural cells expressing the class 1 glucose transporter (GLUT-1) [50]. The size used to define hyperplasia was the same as in the diseased zone, i.. 40 μm. The size of the hyperplastic nerve threads in the transition zone varied from 12 to 64 μm, with an average of 30 μm, which is below the average of 40 μm observed in the diseased zone, with a significant difference [44]. This is in agreement with other studies, which conclude that nerve hyperplasia tends to fade as one approaches the healthy zone [45].

Figure 18 summarises the appearance of CGs and regression of nerve net hyperplasia.

along the transition zone.

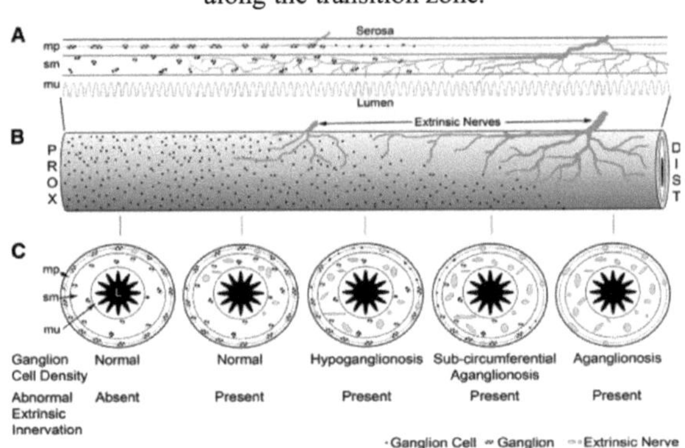

Figure 18: Diagram of the transition zone illustrating the distribution of GCs and extrinsic innervation from the proximal colon to the distal aganglionic segment [50].

(A) Longitudinal section of the entire colonic wall, along the transition zone.

(C) Cross-sections at different sites along the segment of intestine illustrated in (B) to show the circumferential and partial nature of the distribution of GCs and hyperplasia of the extrinsic nerve threads along the transition zone.

8.3.3.3. Other criteria

The presence of GCs alone in the transition zone does not imply normal innervation and therefore does not allow a return to adequate colonic motor function [53]. Other histological lesions are associated, including gangliosclerosis, which is defined by dense hyaline fibrosis surrounding and dissecting the nerve threads of Auerbach's plexuses (Figure 19) [51]. This is the sign most frequently reported the various studies of the transition zone [45,48,50,51]. In Kapur's series, gangliosclerosis was more frequent in older children. However, this sign is not specific to HD since it observed in distended colonic areas sampled from patients with colonic myopathy [45,51]. Other histological criteria that may help to identify the transition zone include hyepreosinophilia around Auerbach's plexuses, and disruption of Cajal's interstitial cells and neurotransmitters. However, most of these criteria are not specific and are inconsistent in the transition zone [51].

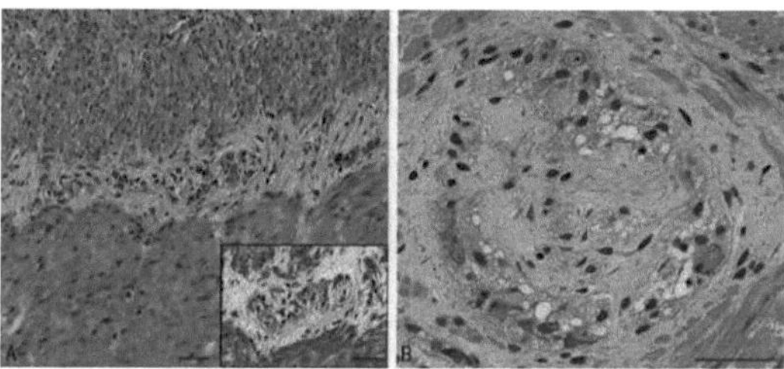

Figure 19: Gangliosclerosis

*(A)*Meyenteric nerve fillet surrounded by an expansive fibrosis better visualised by staining with Masson's Trichrome.

*(B)*More advanced gangliosclerosis with dissecting fibrosis of the nerve nets [51].

8.3.4. Histopathological study of hematein and eosin slides of biopsies taken from diseased areas

The absence of GC is essential to confirm the diagnosis of HD. This sign was observed in 100% of pre-operative biopsies and in 88.6% of intra-operative biopsies taken in the MPA. Nerve hyperplasia is the only positive sign for the diagnosis of HD [44]. In our study, MPA nerve threads were hyperplastic in 100% of preoperative biopsies and in 79% of extemporaneous biopsies. The nerve hyperplasia tends to fade as approaches the healthy zone [45]. The number of hyperplastic nerve threads required for a diagnosis of HD is still debated. While some authors accept nerve hyperplasia in the presence of a single hyperplastic mesh, others require two [45,51]. In extensive forms, nerve hyperplasia is less frequent, both in the transition zone and in the diseased zone [51].

8.4. Extemporaneous examination

Extemporaneous examination is essential in management of HD. It can be carried out in two circumstances:

- Establishing the diagnosis of MH [51]
- Identification of the healthy zone during endoanal resection [3].

Circumferential biopsies are increasingly recommended [45,51]. In our study, 75% of our population had undergone an extemporaneous examination with a concordance rate with the definitive examination of 98%. Only one discordant case was noted in an 8-year-old girl. The result was delayed in one case. The rate of discrepancy between the extemporaneous result and the final result in our study is similar to that reported in the literature, where the rate varies between 1 and 3% [42,46]. Errors occur more frequently in neonates and in biopsies performed for diagnostic purposes [42,52]. The concordance rate was 67% for diagnostic biopsies and 87% for all biopsies combined [52]. Discrepancies are explained by cryopreservation artefacts, the superficial nature of biopsies, the immaturity of GCs and interpretation errors made inexperienced pathologists [42]. The study of acetylcholinesterase activity in its accelerated form can improve the specificity of the extemporaneous examination [51].In the study by Katayoun et al, the consequences of discrepancies during extemporaneous examinations were clinically significant in 1.5% of cases [51]. The case of discrepancy observed in our study led to emergency surgery due to the reappearance of an occlusive syndorme. The clinical consequences are all the more serious when the extemporaneous examination is carried out for diagnostic purposes [42]. Extemporaneous examinations for diagnostic purposes are therefore not recommended [52].

9. STUDY IMMUNOHISTOCHEMISTRY WITH ANTIBODY ANTI-CALRETININ

9.1. CALRETININ

Calretinin is a vitamin D-dependent protein that binds and buffers calcium in nerve fibres. Its absence leads to the accumulation of calcium in intra-cytoplasmic cells, resulting in hyperexcitability and cell degeneration [14]. It is expressed physiologically in several human tissue cells, particularly in the central and peripheral nervous system (neurons, Purkinje cells and astrocytes), luteinised thecal cells of the ovary, Leydig cells and in the adrenal cortex [53].It is most often used in tumour pathology, mainly in the identification of mesothelial tumours. Its expression in other tumours, notably cardiac myxoma, Leydig cell tumours and Merckel's carcinoma has been reported [53].In 2004, Barschak et al. associated the loss of calretinin expression with the absence of CG, a characteristic lesion in HD [15]. Its use for diagnostic purposes in HD has since been the subject of numerous studies [14,37,44,49]. Immunostaining with anti-calretinin antibody results in positivity of CGs and interstitial nerve fibres in the chorion, muscularis mucosae and submucosa [7,13,14]. In our study, identical labelling was observed in all biopsies taken from healthy areas in patients with and without HD.

9.1.1. Calretinin expression profile in the healthy zone

9.1.1.1. Expression of calretinin by ganglion cells

Anti-calretinin antibody is the most commonly used antibody in paediatric gastroenterology laboratories [7,13,14].

Expression calretinin in GCs results in nuclear and cytoplasmic chromogenic deposition [15]. This type of marking was observed in our study in all cases where GCs were positive. In the majority of studies [10,12,38,44], expression of calretinin by GCs is observed in 100% of rectal biopsies taken from patients free of HD. For Holland et al, GCs expressed calretinin in only 16/23 of biopsies taken in healthy areas (70%). In our study, they were labelled in 88% of samples taken in SPAs. absence of labelling could simply reflect the absence of GCs on the section level studied. In the latest recommendations published in 2009, the International Society of Gastroenterology introduced the immunohistochemical study with the anti-calretinin antibody as one of the means of diagnosing HD, but retained only the labelling of GCs as the sole criterion for the positivity of this immunohistochemical test [13]. The evaluation of GC positivity by calretinin alone, as a diagnostic criterion, as suggested by the 2009 recommendations, would therefore offer no advantage over histological examination with haematein-eosin.

9.1.1.2. Expression of calretinin by nerve nets

Associated labelling of the nerve threads, Meissner's and Auerbach's plexuses, was observed in our study. This was also observed in all GC-positive rectal biopsies in other studies [14,54]. Expression of calretinin by nerve threads is common to diseased, transitional and healthy areas [10,14]. The diagnostic value of this labelling is therefore highly contentious, although some authors consider this positivity to be a sufficient criterion for eliminating the diagnosis of MH [10,35]. For Kapur et al, this positivity is observed in extrinsic nerve nets and should therefore not be included as an evaluation criterion in HD [7].

9.1.1.3. Expression of calretin by interstitial nerve fibres

Calretinin is expressed by interstitial nerve fibres in the chorion, tunica muscularis mucosa and submucosa [55]. Labelling of nerve fibres interstitial anti-calretinin antibody is observed in samples taken from healthy areas in subjects with HD. This is identical to that observed in subjects without HD [6,10,43,53]. The expression of calretinin by interstitial nerve fibres has been observed in numerous studies [14,36,37,54,55,55]. It is observed even the absence CG in the nerve nets [54,55]. In our study, interstitial nerve fibres were observed in 91% of samples taken [14,36] in SPAs. The prevalence of this positivity in the various studies varies from 83 to 100% [14,36]. However, the labelling of interstitial nerve fibres is not constant in all layers of the colonic wall. For Haradifar et al, these fibres were more frequently observed in the submucosa (100%), then in the muscular mucosa (90%) and finally in the chorion (70%) in 50 rectal biopsies taken in healthy areas [36].

In our study, labelling was more frequent in the chorion and muscularis mucosae (91%) than in the submucosa (87%). Our results were consistent with those of Yang et al. who observed consistent labelling of interstitial nerve fibres in the chorion and muscularis mucosae in 20 rectal biopsies from patients free of HD [37].

The positivity of interstitial nerve fibres in the chorion is essential, particularly in superficial preoperative rectal biopsies which only include the mucosa. This would make it possible to highlight the innervation of the chorion and muscularis mucosae without necessarily objectifying the CG of the submucosa [11]. This would reduce the number of inconclusive biopsies and the complications of repeat biopsies. Indeed, in an initial study of 17 biopsies deemed inadequate due to a lack of submucosa, the diagnosis of MH was invalidated the positivity of interstitial nerve fibres in the chorion, in concordance with the result of a new biopsy [11]. Labelling with the anti-calretinin antibody allowed the diagnosis of MH to be invalidated in 4 cases of false positives, whose initial diagnosis had been made on histological study with haematein-eosin in association with enzyme-linked immunosorbent assay of acetylcholinesterase activity and immunohistochemical study with S100 protein and neuron-specific enolase (NSE) [4,12,14].

However, all these studies were carried out on a small sample of samples. In our study, all the biopsies received were surgical biopsies. The evaluation of the value of calretinin in superficial rectal biopsies using Noblett forceps was not based on a large sample. therefore not possible. However, the high prevalence of positivity of interstitial nerve fibres in the chorion (91%) in ZPS suggests good results should the Noblett forceps be introduced in the paediatric surgery department of Habib Thameur Hospital. The intensity of labelling of interstitial nerve fibres by the anti-calretinin antibody was high in most studies [10,44,55]. Other studies showed weak to moderate intensity of labelling [12,14]. Weak and discontinuous labelling of interstitial nerve fibres has been sufficient to rule out the diagnosis of MH in some studies. However, this associated with a higher rate of inter-observer discordance and false positives [12,14].

In the Holland et al. study, the prevalence of labelled interstitial nerve fibres increased from

83% to 100% after rereading the slides and collegiate concertation of cases showing low interstitial nerve fibre positivity and which were therefore the source of false positives [14].

9.1.2. Expression of calretnin in the transition zone

Few studies have assessed calretinin expression in the transition zone. Most of the studies carried out have been retrospective and have involved small sample sizes. The methods used to select samples from the transition zone have not always been specified [51,55]. The lack of interest in the study of anti-calretinin antibodies in the transition zone may be explained by the inapplicability of immunohistochemical studies during extemporaneous examinations. As a result, its expression in the transition zone is still poorly defined.

Of the 16 samples taken in the transition zone and included in our immunohistochemical study, calretinin expression showed the presence of CG and interstitial nerve fibres in 63% of cases (10/16 samples). For Kannaiyan et al, expression of calretinin in the transition zone was observed in 83.2% of CGs and 91.6% of hyperplastic nerve nets. Labelling of interstitial nerve fibres with the anti-calretinin antibody was not described in this study [56].

Calretinin expression in the transition zone were as follows: the interstitial nerve fibres of the mucosa appear first, followed by the CG of Meissner plexuses and then those of Auerbach plexuses [10,15,44,54-56,56,57]. However, these data remain unreliable given the small size of the samples studied.

9.1.3. Expression of calretnin in diseased areas

Our results showed a complete absence of anti-calretinin antibody labelling at the level of the diseased zone in 96% of samples for CGs and in 93% of samples for interstitial nerve fibres in patients with MH. CG labelling was observed in the MPAs of 2 patients with HD (4%). Interstitial nerve fibres were labelled in 3 biopsies (7%). The results observed during the immunohistochemical study with the anti-calretinin antibody in biopsies taken in the MPA were similar to many studies found in the literature [10,15,44,54-56,56,57]. There is no anti-calretinin antibody labelling of colonic biopsies for any type of sample taken in a diseased area [6,53]. Mesothelial cells or mast cells are the only cells that can be labelled in the diseased zone in a subject with HD. In the latter case, this positivity is only cytoplasmic and should not be confused with the labelling of interstitial nerve fibres or CGs, and serves as an internal control [14].The absence of labelling of interstitial nerve fibres is thought to be an indicator of aganglionosis [15]. The disappearance of labelling of interstitial nerve fibres concerns the submucosa as well as the muscularis mucosa and the chorion, and its prevalence is very high in samples taken in diseased areas from patients with HD. Numerous authors have reported a 100% absence of labelling of these fibres in rectal biopsies from patients with HD [10,12]. This criterion would therefore be as sensitive as the absence of GC, and would be particularly useful in superficial biopsies. There has been little evaluation of the specificity of this sign. While Holland et al. consider this sign to be pathognomonic of HD [14], other authors have also reported it in the spastic areas of 45 cases of chronic obstructive bowel disease other than HD, notably neurogangliomatosis and intestinal neuronal dysplasia [58].The results concerning the labelling of hyperplastic nerve threads by the anti-calretinin antibody are contradictory in the literature [14]. However, the samples studied were often small and the number of positive cases was low.

10. Study of the diagnostic performance of immunohistochemical study with the anti-calretinin antibody

Pathological examination of rectal biopsies is a cornerstone of HD diagnosis. However, assessment of these biopsies by histological examination using haematein-eosin is fraught with interpretation difficulties due to the immaturity of the GC in premature babies and the superficial nature of some biopsies. It also represents a real time constraint due to the many levels of sectioning required. The study of acetylcholinesterase activity is an undeniable aid in the diagnosis of MH, with specificity close to 100% [10,54-57]. However, its use remains the monopoly of certain specialist centres due to the technical obstacles and difficulties in interpreting this method. Over the last two decades, many authors have focused on the immunohistochemical study of rectal biopsies as a possible solution [15,55,57].

In our study, the sensitivity, specificity, positive predictive value and negative predictive value of the anti-calretinin antibody in the diagnosis of HD were 93%, 100%, 100% and 70% respectively, with good agreement (K=0.791). A total of 3 false negatives were noted. No false positives were observed in our study.

Our results are in line with those in the literature [10,14,55,56]. Some studies show that calretinin is more specific than sensitive. Specificity varies from 80 to 100%, whereas sensitivity ranges from 78 to 100% [10,14,44,55,56]. In the various studies carried out, the reference diagnostic test used varied and the number of samples taken was often limited. Some studies used the enzyme-linked immunosorbent assay of acetylcholinesterase as the reference diagnostic test [38,54,59], while others on a histological study using haematein-eosin [37] or both. In our study, the reference diagnostic method was standard haematein and eosin histopathology.Yang et al sought to compare the diagnostic performance of the anti-calretinin antibody with that of the haematein-eosin histological study. Their study involved 52 superficial rectal biopsies taken with Noblett forceps, 37 of which were taken from patients with MH. Discordance between the standard histological study and the immunohistochemical study was observed in 11 cases (21.1%). They corresponded 11 false positive results, established on histopathological study with haematein eosin and leading to two unnecessary operations. The diagnosis was rectified thanks to the anti-calretinin antibody in all cases [37].

Barschak et al. observed perfect diagnostic concordance of the anti-calretinin antibody with histopathological examination using haematein-eosin. The material included both superficial rectal biopsies and resection specimens. However, the study population was small [15].

Similar results were observed by Hiradfar et al. on 30 biopsies taken from healthy areas and 30 biopsies from diseased areas, with specificity of 100% and sensitivity of 93.3% [36].

For Hollande et al, the association between calretinin expression and the presence or absence of disease was significant ($p<.0001$). Sensitivity was 100% and specificity 83%. In this study, the diagnosis was only made if there was perfect agreement between 3 readers, which explains the low specificity observed [14].

The diagnostic performance of the anti-calretinin antibody observed in the different studies was high independently of the pathologists' level of experience. However, a slight decrease in this performance was quite often noted in young pathologists [15,60]. The main causes of false-negative calretinin antibody immunohistochemistry reported in the literature were short forms of MH which can show labelling of interstitial nerve fibres in the chorion, weak and granular labelling of certain hyperplastic nerve threads and technical problems such as antibody spillage [10,60-62]. One of the 3 false negatives in our study was a short form of MH. The 3 false negatives in our study showed anti-calretinin antibody labelling of CGs and interstitial nerve fibres in two cases and only labelling of interstitial nerve fibres in one case. These false negatives could be explained by sampling in the transition zone. The false positives observed in the literature have been linked to altered expression of calretinin in cryofixed biopsies [10,61]. This has in fact been reported in some studies on samples which have cryofixation. These authors looked at the reliability of calretinin and type 2 microtubule-associated proteins (MAP-2) samples embedded in paraffin after extemporaneous examination. Seventeen biopsies from healthy areas were retrospectively collected, resulting in 6 positive biopsies and seven inconclusive biopsies after immunohistochemical study with anti-calretinin antibody. MAP-2 immunostaining was preserved. This difference remains unexplained [37]. The degree of fixation of the samples is a hypothesis that remains to be explored. In our series, we did not note any false positives.While calretinin has a better diagnostic performance than standard histological examination with haematein-eosin, the comparison of the diagnostic performance of calretinin and acetylcholinesterase is more mixed. The enzyme-linked immunosorbent assay with acetylcholinesterase showed better diagnostic concordance, estimated at 93.5%, compared with only 90.5% for the anti-calretinin antibody. However, the sensitivity of calretinin was much higher, estimated at 100%. Calretinin was able to establish the diagnosis of MH in all inconclusive cases and false negatives found with acetylcholinesterase. The sensitivity and specificity obtained after combining these two methods was 100% [35].In another study, the diagnostic performance of the anti-calretinin antibody was compared with that of standard methods, combining a histological study with haematein-eosin and a study of acetylcholinesterase activity. Calretinin was used to establish the correct diagnosis in all cases. No false positives were observed. Only one false negative was reported due to a low level of hyperplastic nerve net positivity. The concordance rate of the anti-calretinin antibody with post-operative follow-up was high, whereas agreement with standard diagnostic method using acetylcholinesterase and haematein-eosin was only good [10].

In addition to being more sensitive than acetylcholinesterase, calretinin has been shown in various studies to be a more reproducible diagnostic method. The inter-observer reproducibility of the anti-calretinin antibody is better than that of acetylcholinesterase [41].

The diagnostic performance of the anti-calretinin antibody, its accessibility and its common use in other pathologies have led many laboratories to abandon the acetylcholinesterase immuno-enzymatic method [53]. In the light of this work, preoperative biopsies are the reference diagnostic method for HD. These must comply with the quality standards established by the International Society of Gastroenterology in 2009. The immunohistochemical study with anti-calretinin anticoprs is a diagnostic method with sensitivity, specificity and high reproducibility. Marking of interstitial nerve fibres is a reliable criterion and is particularly useful in superficial rectal biopsies. False negatives are associated with short forms of MH, or with low-intensity labelling of interstitial nerve fibres. False positives are associated with altered antigenic expression of calretinin. We therefore recommend the systematic use of an immunohistochemical study with anti-calretinin anticoprs in the absence of CG visualisers, rather than a histopathological study with haematein-eosin in the case of serious therapeutic complications in this disease.

CONCLUSIONS

MH is a congenital disease defined by the absence of CG at the level of Auerbach's and Meissner's plexuses in a more or less extensive part of the digestive tract. It is a rare disease, with a neonatal onset and a mortality rate of 3%. Histopathological examination using haematein-eosin is essential for diagnosing this disease and identifying its extent. In Tunisia, it is the only diagnostic method available in our Pathological Anatomy and Cytology laboratories. In western referral centres, it is combined with enzyme-linked immunosorbent assays of acetylcholinesterase activity compensate for its sensitivity, which varies from 74% to 95%, results in 17% of cases, and delays in diagnosis due to technical constraints requiring several levels of sectioning. Several studies are currently being carried out on biomarkers of HD, in particular on calretinin, a vitamin D-dependent protein that binds and buffers intracellular calcium and is one of the markers of the enteral nervous system.

The aim of this study was to evaluate the diagnostic performance of the anti-calretinin antibody on biopsy samples taken in cases of suspected MH.

We conducted a retrospective study of all biopsies sent to the Department of Pathological Anatomy and Cytology at Habib Thameur Hospital for suspected MH over a period of 22 years (between 1995 and 2017). We first re-read the biopsies, taking into account the sampling area. The results of the rereading were used as a reference test to study the diagnostic performance of the anti-calretinin antibody. Labelling of CGs and/or interstitial nerve fibres present in the chorion, muscularis mucosae or submucosa by the anti-calretinin antibody was retained as a criterion of positivity.

total of 143 samples were collected. These samples were divided into 38 preoperative biopsies and 105 intraoperative biopsies for extemporaneous examination. All preoperative biopsies were surgical, performed under general anaesthesia due to the unavailability of Noblett forceps in the paediatric surgery department of Habib Thameur Hospital. Although superficial rectal biopsies are associated with a low rate of complications, of the order of 0.2%, they are responsible for 17% of inconclusive results due to the small size of the samples, which taken only from the mucosa and submucosa. It is the gold standard diagnostic technique, with diagnostic evidence of level C in the taxonomy of recommendations, subject to meeting the recommendations of the International Society of Gastroenterology, which stipulate that two biopsies of 3 mm each should be taken, including the mucosa and submucosa more than 3 cm from the anal margin, and then correctly embedded in paraffin. In our study, although all biopsies were surgical, only 76% of preoperative biopsies and 89% of intraoperative biopsies for extemporaneous examination involved the entire colonic wall. In 3% of cases, only the mucosa and submucosa were present, probably due to poor orientation of the sample before inclusion in paraffin and a reduced number of section levels.

Histological examination using haematein-eosin is the reference diagnostic method. However, its diagnostic performance is controversial, and essentially depends on the number of sections taken. The diagnostic accuracy of the haematein-eosin study varies between 78.3 and 95%. Combining haematein-eosin histology with acetylcholinesterase enzyme-linked immunosorbent assay or immunohistochemistry increases the diagnostic accuracy to 99.7%. In our study, 87% of preoperative biopsies were examined on a single slice level. The number of cut levels in the literature varied from one reference centre to another, only 33/88 centres performing more than one cut level per sample. The International Committee of Gastroenterology currently recommends that 50 to 75 cut levels be performed and analysed initially, and that other levels be repeated if GCs are not identified.

The rate of discordance between the results of the extemporaneous examination and final examination was 2%. This rate varied from 1 to 3% in the literature. The discrepancies observed were explained by cryopreservation artefacts, the superficial nature of the biopsies, the immaturity of the GCs and interpretation errors made by inexperienced pathologists.

The results of the re-reading were consistent in all cases with the initial results concerning the presence of CG, for both pre-operative and intraoperative biopsies. Discordance in the assessment of nerve net hyperplasia was observed in 7 cases (7%) for intraoperative biopsies. Biopsies taken in the MPA in patients with MH showed a total absence of CG in all preoperative biopsies and in 97% (34/35 cases) of intraoperative biopsies analysed during the extemporaneous examination. The nerve threads were hyperplastic in ZPM in all the preoperative biopsies and in 79% of the intraoperative biopsies and in 68% of the biopsies taken during extemporaneous examination. ZPT. In the literature, nerve threads are considered hyperplastic from a size of 40 µm. Nerve hyperplasia tends to diminish as it approaches the healthy zone and is less frequently observed in extensive forms. Very few studies have examined the prevalence, sensitivity and specificity of nerve hyperplasia in the diagnosis of HD, particularly in the transition zone. Identification of the transition zone during extemporaneous examination is nevertheless essential to avoid persistent severe colonic disorders, which are observed in 34.4% of cases of resections performed in the transition zone or diseased zone. Intraoperative circumferential colonic biopsies are standard practice in many referral centres. The histopathological study of intraoperative circumferential biopsies in the transition zones revealed the presence of aganglionic zones in at least 1/8 of the colonic circumference. The immunohistochemical study with the anti-calretinin antibody involved 110 biopsies.belonging to 68 patients, 60 of whom were MH carriers.

The immunohistochemical study carried out in the SPAs showed identical staining to that seen in patients without MH in the biopsies taken in the MPAs. This labelling took the form of a brown chromogenic deposit, both cytoplasmic and nuclear, in the GCs and granular labelling of the interstitial nerve fibres. It was constantly associated with marking of the nerve threads. The prevalence of calretinin-expressing GCs in the literature ranged from 70 to 100%. The absence of labelling could simply reflect the absence of CGs on the slice level examined. Labelling of interstitial nerve fibres varies from 80 to 100%. This was independent of the cut level. In our study, as in the literature, these were more frequently observed in the chorion and muscularis mucosae. Our results showed a total absence calretinin expression by GCs in the diseased area in 96% of samples and by interstitial nerve fibres in 93% of samples taken from patients with HD. Studies using the anti-calretinin antibody consistently show the absence of any labelling in any sample taken from the diseased area. Mast cells and mesothelial cells are among the only cells that can be labelled in the diseased zone in a subject with HD. The absence of labelling of interstitial nerve fibres has been considered by several authors as an indicator of aganglionosis. The evaluation, as a diagnostic criterion, of calretinin expression alone by GCs, such as suggested by the 2009 guidelines of the International Society of Gastroenterology, offers no more advantages than standard histological examination with haematein-eosin. In the literature, the disappearance of interstitial nerve fibre marking concerns the submucosa, the muscularis mucosa and the chorion, and is observed in up to 100% of rectal biopsies from patients with HD. The absence of labelling of interstitial nerve fibres would be particularly important during examination of superficial rectal biopsies.

In the literature, the results concerning the marking of nerve nets are contradictory. In fact, this is observed in diseased areas, healthy areas and transitional areas. Some authors believe that extrinsic nerve nets also express calretinin and should therefore not be included in the criteria for evaluating HD. In our study, the sensitivity, specificity, positive predictive value and negative predictive value of calretinin in the diagnosis of HD were 93%, 100%, 100% and 70% respectively, with good agreement (K=0.791). Calretinin is more specific than sensitive, with specificity ranging from 95 to 100% and sensitivity from 78 to 97.6%. The literature review shows a better diagnostic performance of the anti-calretinin antibody compared with haematein-eosin staining. However, the comparison between the diagnostic performance of the anti-calretinin antibody and the enzyme-linked immunosorbent assay of acetylcholinesterase is more mixed. For some authors, the acetylcholinesterase enzyme-linked immunosorbent assay has better specificity than calretinin, estimated at 93.5% compared with 90.5% for calretinin. However, the sensitivity of calretinin was much higher, estimated at 100%. Calretinin was able to establish the diagnosis of MH in all biopsies with inconclusive results during the acetylcholinesterase enzyme-linked immunosorbent assay. The sensitivity and specificity obtained by combining these two methods was 100%. A total of three false negatives were identified. No false positives were reported using the results of the haematein-eosin histology study as the reference diagnostic test. The causes of false negatives reported in the literature are short forms of MH which can show the presence of interstitial nerve fibres in the chorion, weak and granular marking of certain hyperplastic nerve nets and technical problems such as antibody overflow. The false negatives observed in our study could be explained by sampling in the transition zone. A defect It is possible that the haematein-eosin test was performed on a single level of section. However, the good clinical course observed and the presence of pathological and healthy margins on the surgical specimen contradict this hypothesis. The false positives observed in the literature are explained by an alteration in expression of of calretinin on cryopreserved biopsies. The retrospective nature of our study, the small sample size, and the absence of biopsies were the main limitations of our study. Preoperative biopsies are the reference diagnostic method for HD. These must comply with the quality standards established by the International Society of Gastroenterology in 2009. Unlike the labelling of nerve fibres, the labelling of interstitial nerve fibres is a reliable and sufficient criterion for anti-calretinin antibody positivity. The systematic use of an immunohistochemical study with anti-calretinin antibody in the absence of CG visualisation on histopathological study with haematein-eosin is a reasonable alternative given the serious therapeutic implications of this disease.

REFERENCES

[1]Martucciello G. Hirschsprung's disease, one of the most difficult diagnoses in pediatric surgery: a review of the problems from clinical practice to the bench. Eur J Pediatr Surg.2008;18(3):140-9.

[2]Löf Granström A. Wester T. Mortality in swedish patients with Hirschsprung disease. Pediatr Surg Int. 2017; 33(11): 1177-81.

[3]Hervieux E. Place de l'examen extemporané dans la prise en charge de la forme recto sigmoïdienne de la maladie de Hirschsprung. Henri Warembourg Faculty of Medicine. 2013.

[4]Bhatnagar SN. Hirschsprung's disease in newborns. J Neonatal Surg 2013;2(4): 51.

[5]Fkih A. Interest of imaging in the diagnosis Hirschprung's disease.Faculté de Medécine de Monastir 2014.

[6]Peyvasteh M, Askapour S, Ostadian N, Moghimi M-R, Javaherizadeh H. Diagnostic accuracy of barium enema findings in Hirschsprung's disease. Arq Bras Cir Dig 2016;29:155-8.

[7]Kapur RP. Practical pathology and genetics of Hirschsprung's disease. Semin Pediatr Surg 2009;18(4):212-23.

[8]De Haro Jorge I, Palazón Bellver P, Julia Masip V, Saura García L, Ribalta Farres T, Cuadras Pallejà D, et al. Effectiveness of calretinin and role of age in the diagnosis of Hirschsprung disease. Pediatr Surg Int 2016;32:723-7.

[9]Pacheco MC, Bove KE. Variability of acetylcholinesterase hyperinnervation patterns in distal rectal suction biopsy specimens in Hirschsprung disease. Pediatric and Developmental Pathology 2008;11:274-82.

[10]Guinard-Samuel V, Bonnard A, de Lagausie P, Philippe-Chomette P, Alberti C, El Ghoneimi A, et al. Calretinin immunohistochemistry: a simple and efficient tool to diagnose Hirschsprung disease. Mod Pathol. 2009;22:1379-84.

[11]Gonzalo DH, Plesec T. Hirschsprung disease and use of calretinin in inadequate rectal suction biopsies. Arch Pathol Lab Med 2013;137:1099-102.

[12]Cinel L, Ceyran B, Güçlüer B. Calretinin immunohistochemistry for the diagnosis of Hirschprung disease in rectal biopsies. Pathol Res Pract 2015;211:50-4.

[13] Knowles CH, de Giorgio R, Kapur RP, Bruder E, Farrugia G, Geboes K, et al. Gastrointestinal neuromuscular pathology: Guidelines for histological techniques and reporting on behalf of the gastro 2009 international working group. Acta Neuropathol 2009;118:271-301.

[14] Holland SK, Ramalingam P, Podolsky RH, Reid-Nicholson MD, Lee JR. Calretinin immunostaining as an adjunct in the diagnosis of Hirschsprung disease. Annals of Diagnostic Pathol 2011;15:323-8.

[15] Barshack I, Fridman E, Goldberg I, Chowers Y, Kopolovic J. The loss of calretinin expression indicates aganglionosis in Hirschsprung's disease. J Clin Pathol. 2004;57(7):712-6.

[16] Serafini S, Santos MM, Aoun Tannuri AC, Zerbini MCN, de Mendonça Coelho MC, de Oliveira Gonçalves J, et al. Is hematoxylin-eosin staining in rectal mucosal and submucosal biopsies still useful for the diagnosis of Hirschsprung disease.Diagn Pathol. 2017;12(1):84.

[17] Stocker S, Dehner L. Stocker and Dehner's Pediatric Pathology. 3rd edition Alphen aan den Rijn,Wolters kluwer, 2010.

[18] Harrison MW, Deltz DM, Campbell JR, Campbell TJ. Diagnosis and management of hirschsprung's disease. Am J Surg 1986;152:49-56.

[19] EL Ghouzi S. Hirschsprung's disease in older children about 16 cases. Université Cadi Ayyad Faculté de Médécine et de Pharmacie Marrakech. 2013.

[20] Núñez-Ramos R, Fernández RM, González-Velasco M, Ruiz-Contreras J, Galán-Gómez E, Núñez-Núñez R, et al. A scoring system to predict the severity of Hirschsprung disease at diagnosis and its correlation with molecular genetics. Pediatric and Developmental Pathology 2017;20(1) 28-37.

[21] Ikeda K, Goto S. Diagnosis and treatment of Hirschsprung's disease in japan: an analysis of 1628 patients. Ann Surg 1984;199:400-5.

[22] Weitzman JJ, Hanson BA, Brennan LP. Management of Hirschsprung's disease with the swenson procedure. J Pediatr Surg 1972;7:157-62.

[23] Menezes M, Corbally M, Puri P. Long-term results of bowel function after treatment for Hirschsprung's disease: a 29-year review. Pediatr Surg Int 2006;22:987-90.

[24] Philippe-Chomette P, Peuchmaur M, Aigrain Y. Hirschsprung's disease children Diagnosis and management. Journal de Pédiatrie et de Puériculture 2008;21:1-12.

[25] Ellahya H. Hirschsprung's disease in older children: A propos de 43 cas. Cadi Ayyad University, Faculty of Medicine and Pharmacy, Marrakech. 2011.

[26] Essghir A. Hirschsprung's disease adults: 16 cases. Faculty Medicine of Monastir. 2010.

[27] Moore SW, Zaahl M. Segmental aganglionosis (zonal aganglionosis or "skip" lesions) in Hirschsprungs disease: a report of 2 unusual cases. J Pediatr Surg 2013;5:495-500.

[28] Tlili S. Hirschsprung's disease: Therapeutic news: About 43 cases. Tunis Faculty of Medicine. 2013.

[29] Moore SW, Zaahl M. Total colonic aganglionosis and Hirschsprung's disease: a review. J Pediatr Surg 2015;31:1-9.

[30] Ax SÖ, Arnbjörnsson E, Gisselsson-Nord D. A comparison of rectal suction and full Wall biopsy in Hirschsprung's disease. Surg Science 2014;05:15-9.

[31] Muise ED, Cowles RA. Rectal biopsy for Hirschsprung's disease: A review of techniques, pathology, and complications. World J Pediatr 2016;12(2):135-41.

[32] de Lorijn F, Kremer LCM, Reitsma JB, Benninga MA. Diagnostic tests in Hirschsprung disease: A systematic review. J Pediatr Gastroenterol Nutr 2006;42:496-505.

[33] de Lorijn F, Reitsma JB, Voskuijl WP, Aronson DC, ten Kate FJ, Smets AMJB, et al. Diagnosis of Hirschsprung's disease: a prospective, comparative accuracy study of common tests. J Pediatr 2005;146:787-92.

[34] Szylberg L, Marszalek A. Diagnosis of Hirschsprung's disease with particular emphasis on histopathology: a systematic review of current literature. Przeglad Gastroenterologiczny 2014;9:264-9.

[35] Jeong H, Jung HR, Hwang I, Kwon SY, Choe M, Kang YN, et al. Diagnostic accuracy of combined acetylcholinesterase histochemistry and calretinin immunohistochemistry of rectal biopsy specimens in Hirschsprung's disease. Int J Surg Pathol. 2018;26(6):507- 13.

[36] Hiradfar M, Sharifi N, Khajedaluee M, Zabolinejad N, Taraz Jamshidi S. Calretinin immunohistochemistry: an aid in the diagnosis of Hirschsprung's disease. Iran J Basic Med Sci 2012;15:1053-9.

[37] Yang WI, Oh J-T. Calretinin and microtubule-associated protein-2 (MAP-2) immunohistochemistry in the diagnosis of Hirschsprung's disease. J Pediatr Surg 2013;48:2112-7.

[38] Jiang M, Li K, Li S, Yang L, Yang D, Zhang X, et al. Calretinin, S100 and protein gene

product 9.5 immunostaining of rectal suction biopsies in the diagnosis of Hirschsprung's disease. Am J Transl Res 2016;8(7):3159-68.

[39] Setiadi JA, Dwihantoro A, Iskandar K, Heriyanto DS, Gunadi. The utility of the hematoxylin and eosin staining in patients with suspected Hirschsprung disease. BMC Surg. 2017;17(1):71.

[40] Karim S, Hession C, Marconi S, Gang DL, Otis CN. The identification of ganglion cells in Hirschsprung disease by the immunohistochemical detection of ret oncoprotein. Am J Clin Pathol. 2006;126(1):49-54.

[41] Kapur RP, Raess PW, Hwang S, Winter C. Choline transporter immunohistochemistry: An effective substitute for acetylcholinesterase histochemistry to diagnose Hirschsprung disease with formalin-fixed paraffin-embedded rectal biopsies. Pediatric and Developmental Pathology. 2017;20(4):308-20.

[42] Shayan K, Smith C, Langer JC. Reliability of intraoperative frozen sections in the management of Hirschsprung's disease. J Pediatr Surg. 2004;39(9):1345-8.

[43] Burki T, Kiho L, Scheimberg I, Phelps S, Misra D, Ward H, et al. Neonatal functional intestinal obstruction and the presence of severely immature ganglion cells on rectal biopsy: 6 year experience. Pediatr Surg Int 2011;27:487-90.

[44] Volpe A, Alaggio R, Midrio P, Iaria L, Gamba P. Calretinin, b-tubulin immunohistochemistry, and submucosal nerve trunks morphology in Hirschsprung disease: possible applications in clinical practice. J Pediatr Gastroenterol Nutr 2013;57:780-7.

[45] Coe A, Collins MH, Lawal T, Louden E, Levitt MA, Peña A. Reoperation for Hirschsprung disease: pathology of the resected problematic distal pull-through. Pediatric and Developmental Pathology 2012;15(1):30-8.

[46] Friedmacher F, Puri P. Residual aganglionosis after pull-through operation for Hirschsprung's disease: a systematic review and meta-analysis. Pediatr Surg Int 2011;27:1053-57.

[47] Kapur RP, Kennedy AJ. Histopathologic delineation of the transition zone in short-segment Hirschsprung disease. Pediatric and Developmental Pathology 2013;16:252- 66.

[48] Ghose SI, Squire BR, Stringer MD, Batcup G, Crabbe DC. Hirschsprung's disease: problems with transition-zone pull-through. J Pediatr Surg 2000;35(12):1805-9.

[49] Najjar S, Ahn S, Kasago I, Zuo C, Umrau K, Ainechi S, et al. Image processing and

analysis of mucosal calretinin staining to define the transition zone in Hirschsprungd: a pilot study. Eur J Pediatr Surg2019;29(2):179-87.

[50] Kapur RP, Kennedy AJ. Transitional zone pull through: surgical pathology considerations. Pediatr Surg Int 2012;003-4.

[51] Kapur RP. Histology of the transition zone in Hirschsprung disease. Am J Surg Pathol 2016;40:1637-46.

[52] Maia DM. The reliability of frozen-section diagnosis in the pathologic evaluation of Hirschsprung's disease. Am J Surg Pathol. 2009;33(5):749-58.

[53] Lugli A, Forster Y, Haas P, Nocito A, Bucher C, Bissig H, et al. Calretinin expression in human normal and neoplastic tissues: a tissue microarray analysis on 5233 tissue samples. Hum Pathol. 2003;34:994-1000.

[54] Alexandrescu S, Rosenberg H, Tatevian N. Role of calretinin immunohistochemical stain in evaluation of Hirschsprung disease: an institutional experience. Int J Clin Exp Pathol 2013;6:2955-61.

[55] Kapur RP, Reed RC, Finn LS, Patterson K, Johanson J, Rutledge JC. Calretinin immunohistochemistry versus acetylcholinesterase histochemistry in the evaluation of suction rectal biopsies for Hirschsprung disease. Pediatric and Developmental Pathology 2009;12:6-15.

[56] Kannaiyan L, Madabhushi S, Malleboyina R, Are NK, Reddy KR, Rao B. Calretinin immunohistochemistry: A new cost-effective and easy method for diagnosis of Hirschsprung's disease. J Indian Assoc Pediatr Surg 2013;18(2):66-8.

[57] Morris MI, Soglio DB-D, Ouimet A, Aspirot A, Patey N. A study of calretinin in Hirschsprung pathology, particularly in total colonic aganglionosis. J of Pediat Surg 2013;48:1037-43.

[58] Wang S-Q, Zhu J, Wang Y, Zhao Z-B, Li X-Q, Li S-S, et al. Utilization of RET, Bcl-2 and CR immunohistochemistry in the diagnosis of Hirschsprung disease and its allied disorders. Int J Clin Exp Pathol 2016;9(10):10390-97.

[59] De Arruda Lourenção PLT, Takegawa BK, Ortolan EVP, Terra SA, Rodrigues MAM. A useful panel for the diagnosis of Hirschsprung disease in rectal biopsies: calretinin immunostaining and acetylcholinesterase histochesmistry. Annals of Diagnostic Pathology 2013;17:352-6.

[60] Kacr A, Arikok AT, Azili MN, Ekberli Agirbas G, Tiryaki T. Calretinin immunohistochemistry in Hirschsprung's disease: An adjunct to formalin-based diagnosis. Turk J Gastroenterol 2012;23(3):226-33.

[61] Kok Hing L, Wei Keat W, Tony Kiat L, Alwin Hwai Liang L, Shireen N, Kenneth Tou En CH. Primary diagnosis of Hirschsprung disease: calretinin immunohistochemistry in rectal suction biopsies, with emphasis on diagnostic pitfalls. World J Pathol 2014;3:14- 22.

[62] Chung PHY, Wong KKY, Tam PKH, Leung MWY, Chao NSY, Liu KKW, et al. Are all patients with short segment Hirschsprung's disease equal? A retrospective multicenter study. Ped Surg Int 2018;34:47-53.

DIAGNOSIS OF HIRSCHSPRUNG'S DISEASE: STUDY OF DIAGNOSTIC PERFORMANCE OF THE ANTI-CALRETININ ANTIBODY

SUMMARY

***Introduction**: Hirschsprung's disease (HD) is a rare congenital disorder defined by the absence of ganglion cells (GCs) in a more or less extensive segment of the digestive tract. Its diagnosis in Tunisia is based solely on histopathological study using haematein-eosin, which is a sometimes restrictive technique with a sensitivity ranging from 74 to 90%. Several studies are currently being carried out on biomarkers of HD, in particular on the anti-calretinin antibody.*

***Objective**: To evaluate the diagnostic performance of the anti-calretinin antibody on biopsy samples. carried out in cases of suspected MH.*

***Methods**: This was a retrospective study of all biopsies referred for suspected MH. We reread the slides for haematein-eosin, the results of which were used as the reference diagnostic test in assessing the diagnostic performance of the anti-calretinin antibody.*

***Results**: A total of 80 patients were included, 69 of whom had MH. All pre-operative biopsies were surgical. The results of the re-reading were consistent in all cases with the initial results concerning the presence of CG. Discordance in the assessment of nerve net hyperplasia was observed in 7 cases (7%). Biopsies taken from presumed diseased areas (PDAs) patients with MH showed a complete absence of CGs in all preoperative biopsies and in 97% (34/35 cases) of intraoperative biopsies. The immunohistochemical study using the anti-calretinin antibody in biopsies taken in the presumed healthy zone (PHZ) showed brown chromogenic deposits, both cytoplasmic and nuclear, in the GCs and granular marking of the interstitial nerve fibres. Marking of the nerve threads was constantly associated. This staining was identical to that observed in biopsies taken in MPAs from patients free of MH. In MPA biopsies, interstitial nerve fibres expressed calretinin more frequently (91%) than CGs (89%). In MPA biopsies, CGs were labelled in 2 biopsies while interstitial nerve fibres were labelled in 3 biopsies (7.3%). The sensitivity, specificity, positive predictive value and negative predictive value of the anti-calretinin antibody were 93%, 100%, 100% and 70% respectively, with good agreement (**k=0**.791). In total, we identified three false negatives. No false positives were reported.*

Conclusions: *The immunohistochemical study with the anti-calretinin antibody is a diagnostic tool with high sensitivity, specificity and reproducibility. Labelling of interstitial nerve fibres is a reliable criterion and is particularly useful in superficial rectal biopsies. The systematic use of an immunohistochemical study with the anti-calretinin antibody in the absence of CG visualisation in the histopathological study with haematein-eosin is a reasonable alternative given the serious therapeutic implications of HD.*

KeyWords- Hirschsprung's disease-calretinin-sensitivity-specificity-immunohistochemistry

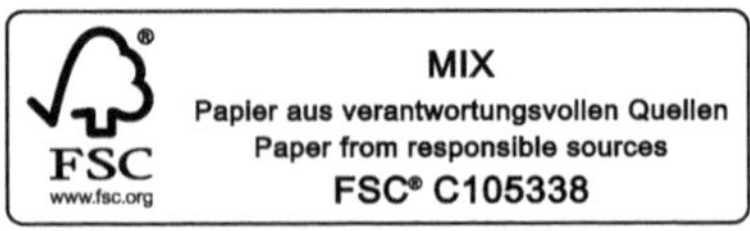

Printed by Books on Demand GmbH, Norderstedt / Germany